BIOTECHNOLOGY
INTELLIGENCE
UNIT

THE SV40 REPLICON MODEL FOR ANALYSIS OF ANTICANCER DRUGS

Robert M. Snapka

Associate Professor of Radiology
The Ohio State University
Columbus, Ohio, U.S.A.

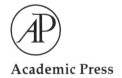

Academic Press

R.G. LANDES COMPANY
AUSTIN

BIOTECHNOLOGY INTELLIGENCE UNIT

THE SV40 REPLICON MODEL FOR ANALYSIS OF ANTICANCER DRUGS

R.G. LANDES COMPANY
Austin, Texas, U.S.A.

This book is printed on acid-free paper.
Copyright 1996 © by R.G. Landes Company and Academic Press, Inc.

Please address all inquiries to the Publisher:
R.G. Landes Company
909 Pine Street, Georgetown, Texas, U.S.A. 78626
Phone: 512/ 863 7762; FAX: 512/ 863 0081

Academic Press, Inc.
525 B Street, Suite 1900, San Diego, California, U.S.A. 92101-4495

United Kingdom Edition published by Academic Press Limited
24-28 Oval Road, London NW1 7DX, United Kingdom

International Standard Book Number (ISBN): 0-12-65360-9

Printed in the United States of America

While the authors, editors and publisher believe that drug selection and dosage and the specifications and usage of equipment and devices, as set forth in this book, are in accord with current recommendations and practice at the time of publication, they make no warranty, expressed or implied, with respect to material described in this book. In view of the ongoing research, equipment development, changes in governmental regulations and the rapid accumulation of information relating to the biomedical sciences, the reader is urged to carefully review and evaluate the information provided herein.

Library of Congress Cataloging-in-Publication Data

The SV40 replicaon model for analysis of anticancer drugs / Robert M. Snapka
     p. cm. — (Biotechnology intelligence unit)
   Includes bibliographical references and index.
   ISBN 0-12-65360-9 (alk. paper)
   1. SV40 (virus). 2. Viral genetics. 3. Antineoplastic agents—Research—Methodology.
4. DNA-drug interactions. I. Title. II. Series.
       [DNLM: 1. Polyomavirus macacae—genetics. 2. Polyomavirus macacae—drug effects. 3. DNA Replication—drug effects. 4. Models, Genetic. QW 165.5.P2 W669s 1996]
QR406.2.S56S64 1996
616.99'4061—dc20
DNLM/DLC
for Library of Congress

96-579
CIP

PUBLISHER'S NOTE

R.G. Landes Company publishes six book series: *Medical Intelligence Unit, Molecular Biology Intelligence Unit, Neuroscience Intelligence Unit, Tissue Engineering Intelligence Unit, Environmental Intelligence Unit* and *Biotechnology Intelligence Unit.* The authors of our books are acknowledged leaders in their fields and the topics are unique. Almost without exception, no other similar books exist on these topics.

Our goal is to publish books in important and rapidly changing areas of bioscience for sophisticated researchers and clinicians. To achieve this goal, we have accelerated our publishing program to conform to the fast pace in which information grows in the biosciences. Most of our books are published within 90 to 120 days of receipt of the manuscript. We would like to thank our readers for their continuing interest and welcome any comments or suggestions they may have for future books.

Deborah Muir Molsberry
Publications Director
R.G. Landes Company

CONTENTS

EDITORS

Robert M. Snapka, Ph.D.
Associate Professor of Radiology
The Ohio State University
Columbus, Ohio, U.S.A.
Chapters 1-6, 8

CONTRIBUTORS

John M. Cassady, Ph.D.
Professor and Dean,
  College of Pharmacy
The Ohio State University
Columbus, Ohio, U.S.A.
Chapter 6

Christopher A. Ferrer, B.S.
Graduate Research Associate,
Department of Medical
  Microbiology
  and Immunology
The Ohio State University
Columbus, Ohio, U.S.A.
Chapter 6

Linda H. Malkas, Ph.D.
Associate Professor,
Department of Pharmacology
University of Maryland School
  of Medicine
Baltimore, Maryland, U.S.A.
Chapter 7

Paskasari A. Permana, Ph.D.
Postdoctoral Fellow
National Institutes of Health
CDNS
Phoenix, Arizona, U.S.A.
Chapter 8

Nan-Jun Sun, B.S.
Professor, Institute
  of Medicinal Plants
Chinese Academy
  of Medical Sciences; and
Vice President, Chinese
  Pharmaceutical Association
China
Chapter 6

Edith F. Yamasaki, M.S.
Research Associate,
Department of Radiology
The Ohio State University
Columbus, Ohio, U.S.A.
Chapter 4

PREFACE

$\int$ ince its discovery as an ominous contaminant of early polio vaccines, simian virus 40 (SV40) has become a powerful research tool. SV40 and the closely related polyomavirus have greatly increased our understanding of carcinogenesis. The product of the p53 tumor suppressor gene which is mutated in so many human cancers was originally discovered as a cellular protein bound to the viral large T antigen. Interactions of this multifunctional viral oncogene with other cellular proteins and with promoter regions of cellular genes are still very active research areas. SV40 is routinely used to transform human cell types in order to immortalize them for continued study.

SV40 has also contributed greatly to our knowledge of DNA replication and chromatin structure in mammalian cells. When it was realized that the virus must make use of host cell DNA replication enzymes and that its DNA is packaged in host-derived histones organized into nucleosomes, the viral chromosome came to be regarded as a "minichromosome" which could serve as a model for mammalian replicons. In comparison to mammalian chromosomes, the SV40 genome has many advantages for studies of DNA replication, including high copy number, known DNA sequence, well mapped genetic elements, easy extractability as chromatin or DNA, uniformity of chromatin structure and ease of handling (without random shearing of the DNA). Many of the techniques used to study DNA replication in mammalian cells become especially powerful when used with SV40 or polyoma. Early studies of SV40 DNA replication and its disruption by treatments such as ultraviolet radiation made use of several types of density gradient ultracentrifugation. However, greatly improved separations of viral DNA replication intermediates are possible with gel electrophoresis—especially two-dimensional gel techniques. High resolution gel electrophoresis was applied to the SV40 DNA replication system by the author to demonstrate that topoisomerase II-targeting drugs such as doxorubicin inhibit chromosome separation and to show that collisions between moving DNA replication forks and camptothecin-stabilized topoisomerase I-DNA complexes result in double strand DNA breaks at the replication forks.

This volume of the *Biotechnology Intelligence Unit* series reviews the history of SV40 as a mammalian replicon model and covers the techniques used to analyze viral DNA replication. Special detail is devoted to the newer high resolution gel electrophoresis techniques. One chapter is devoted to the molecular events of drug-induced DNA replication fork failure and subsequent recombinational events. Other chapters focus on topoisomerase II and the termination of DNA replication, the effects of DNA damaging agents, in vitro SV40 DNA replication systems, drug discovery with SV40 and replication of the SV40 circular oligomers. It is hoped that this volume will be of use to researchers in the areas of DNA replication, DNA repair, experimental cancer chemotherapy, drug discovery and virology.

========= CHAPTER 1 =========

PAPOVAVIRUS MODELS FOR MAMMALIAN REPLICONS

Robert M. Snapka

Simian virus 40 (SV40) and polyomavirus have contributed greatly to our knowledge of cell biology and carcinogenesis. The viral tumor antigens are oncogenes which interact with cellular proteins involved in cell cycle control. These small papovaviruses have contributed to our understanding of DNA replication, transcription and chromatin structure. They have been favorite systems for such studies because of their extensive use of host cell enzymes and proteins and because of their unique advantages as experimental systems. The similarities between papovavirus chromosomes and mammalian chromosomes make them good models for mammalian replicons.

SV40 and polyomavirus are being used with increasing frequency in studies aimed at understanding how anticancer drugs and carcinogens disrupt DNA replication in mammalian cells. This book reviews their use in such studies and provides examples of high-resolution techniques which can be applied to the analysis of drug action. This chapter introduces the papovaviruses and reviews the structure of viral chromatin. Other chapters focus on techniques for analysis of SV40 DNA replication, inactivation of replicating chromosomes by inhibitors of DNA replication enzymes, termination of DNA replication, disruption of DNA replication by DNA damage, in vitro SV40 DNA replication, drug discovery with SV40 and replication of polymeric SV40 genomes.

The SV40 Replicon Model for Analysis of Anticancer Drugs,
edited by Robert M. Snapka. ©1996 R.G. Landes Company.

PAPOVAVIRUSES

The papovaviruses are small, non-enveloped DNA viruses with icosahedral virions composed of 72 capsomers surrounding a circular double strand DNA genome. The virions contain only DNA and protein. There are two papovavirus genera: the papilloma viruses with virions approximately 55 nm in diameter and genomes of about 8,000 bp, and the polyoma viruses with virions about 45 nm in diameter and genomes of about 5,000 bp. The polyoma viruses include SV40 and polyoma, two viruses which have been intensively studied because of their ability to transform cells of many types—the origin of "poly" in the name of the genus. In addition to being useful model systems for the study of carcinogenesis, these viruses have become models for mammalian chromosomes and replicons. The DNA packaged in the virions is associated with host cell-encoded histones which are organized into nucleosomes. More importantly, the replicating viral genomes are organized into chromatin in the cell nucleus. Due to the limited coding capacity of the virus, most of the enzymes needed for replication of the viral genomes are provided by the host cell. The extensive use of host cell DNA replication enzymes and the organization of the viral genomes into "minichromosomes" make them useful models for mammalian replicons. These models offer a number of advantages over cellular chromosomes in the study of DNA replication. Both SV40 and polyoma can be selectively extracted from infected cells as either viral DNA[1] or as viral chromatin, leaving behind the cellular DNA or chromatin. The viral DNA or chromatin can be easily pipetted or manipulated without the random shearing which plagues work with cellular DNA or chromatin. The virus is in high copy number at the peak of DNA replication (over 100,000 copies per infected cell for SV40, but lower for polyoma). The copy number for any particular sequence in mammalian cells (even those with amplified genes) is lower by orders of magnitude. The DNA sequences of both SV40 and polyoma are known, and genetic elements, such as the DNA replication origin, the replication terminus, enhancers and promoters, are all mapped. Since the viral genomes are superhelical DNA circles, they can be used to assay DNA damage that causes DNA strand breaks (nicking) either directly or indirectly. DNA damage that has not caused DNA nicking can also be detected and/or quantitated with DNA damage-specific endonucleases or treatments that cause DNA strand breaks at sites of damage. Finally, the circular DNA chromosomes can reveal their topological history by changes in superhelicity, knotting or catenation. The various replication intermediates and topological forms can be resolved by high resolution one- or two-dimensional gel electrophoresis, by density gradient ultracentrifugation, or by isopycnic banding. Preparation of virus stocks and radiolabeling of viral DNA have been described in detail.[2-6] The biology of SV40 and polyoma has been reviewed by Tooze.[7]

THE SV40 GENOME

The complete DNA sequence of SV40 (strain 776) is known.[7] From the DNA sequence, the size of the genome was determined to be 5,248 bp. Polyoma virus has a slightly larger genome of 5,292 bp.[7] The DNA in virions is in the form of a covalently closed double stranded circle which is underwound. In other words, the DNA strands of the Watson-Crick helix have a linking deficit with respect to linear double strand DNAs or nicked DNA circles. This torsionally stressed, superhelical DNA coils upon itself in solution to form a compact structure, form I DNA. The superhelicity of the viral chromosomes is a reflection of chromatin structure. The structure, replication and transcription of the SV40 genome have been reviewed.[8-11] Chapter 7 covers in vitro SV40 DNA replication and reviews details of the enzymes of DNA replication and the functional elements of the SV40 early region.

SV40 CHROMATIN

In both virions and cells, the viral DNA is associated with cell-derived histones.[12-17] These early studies detected the core histones but did not detect H1 (see below). The histones of the viral nucleoprotein complex are organized into nucleosomes,[18,19] as they are in cellular chromatin. Thus, the SV40 and polyomavirus nucleoprotein complexes are considered minichromosomes. The histones associated with viral DNA are highly acetylated.[20] Acetylation of histones may facilitate transcription.[21] The composition, structure and compactness of viral minichromosomes is determined by the extraction procedure and the composition of buffers in purification.

LINKING NUMBER PARADOX

The number of nucleosomes in an SV40 or polyomavirus minichromosome corresponds to the number of negative superhelical coils in the covalently closed form I DNA after the minichromosome is deproteinized. There is about one negative superhelical coil per nucleosome. This relationship can also be demonstrated with nucleosomes formed on circular DNAs in vitro. The nucleosome core DNA is 146 bp long and is wrapped around the nucleosome 1.8 times in a left handed toroidal helix. Negative superhelicity is a linkage deficit with respect to the linkage of the two strands of the DNA helix in relaxed circular DNA. This difference in linking number between superhelical and relaxed DNA (ΔLk) is distributed between altered helix period or twist (Tw) and writhing of the helix axis (Wr) so that $\Delta Lk = \Delta Tw + \Delta Wr$. The wrapping of DNA around a nucleosome is writhing, and translates into right handed plectonemic supercoiling when the core is removed. In the case of DNA wrapped on nucleosomes, the core is protein, and it can be removed by proteolysis or solvent extraction. Calculations show that the change in linking number due to the wrapping of DNA on nucleosomes should correspond to a linking difference (ΔLk) of -1.38 per nucleosome rather than the experimentally observed value of -1.01.[22] This is the linking number paradox, which can be resolved if higher order chromatin structure or nucleosome stacking contributes a linking difference or if distortions in the shape of the nucleosome twist the DNA.

HISTONE H1

SV40 minichromosomes extracted from infected cells are associated with histone H1 in addition to the other four histones.[23] The ratio of H1 to the other four histones is similar to that in cellular chromatin, and the H1 is associated with internucleosomal linker regions. Addition of histone H1 to purified minichromosomes lacking it causes a striking condensation of the viral chromatin.[24] H1-containing SV40 minichromosomes are compact 300 Å spheres at physiological ionic strength.[25] This condensed form of the minichromosome is very resistant to staphylococcal nuclease, an enzyme that has been used widely to selectively digest the internucleosomal spacer regions of chromatin. The compact form was not resistant to DNase I. Without histone H1 or at other ionic strengths, the viral minichromosome becomes extended and beaded. The condensed H1-associated viral minichromosome has a sedimentation coefficient of 70S.[26-28] At high ionic strength, histone H1 is released, and the minichromosome unfolds to become an extended beads-on-a-string form that sediments at 40S. Re-addition of H1 causes recompaction of the chromosome. SV40 nucleoprotein complexes extracted from infected cells have also been reported to have histone H3 and H4 subfractions differing in levels of acetylation.[29] The viral chromatin is significantly more acetylated than that of the host cell. High mobility group proteins 1 and 2 are found with H1 in previrions.[30] There is evidence that the SV40 origin region is involved in nucleosome assembly in vivo and that H1-nucleosome interactions are important to the assembly process.[31] Physiological amounts of histone H1 do not inhibit DNA replication in an in vitro SV40 DNA replication system, but high levels are inhibitory.[32] SV40 virions have been reported to contain histone H1 in stoichiometric proportions,[33] however, other laboratories have found no H1 in virions.[29,30]

NUCLEOSOME FREE REGION

The first evidence that nucleosomes were unevenly distributed on SV40 minichromosomes came from nuclease digestion studies that indicated increased accessibility in a region around the origin of DNA replication. Varshavsky and coworkers found greatly enhanced cleavage of viral minichromosomes by Bgl I relative to other restriction endonucleases.[34] Since Bgl I cleaves SV40 DNA near the origin of DNA replication, it was suggested that the region is selectively exposed in minichromosomes. Similar results were obtained with both formaldehyde fixed and unfixed chromosomes. Scott and Wigmore found that DNase I selectively digests the origin region of SV40 minichromosomes.[35] They concluded that, in at least part of the population of minichromosomes, a region located between map positions 0.67 and 0.73 is preferentially cleaved by DNase I or by endogenous nuclease, but not by staphylococcal nuclease. Additional experiments indicated that this region was histone-free and unusually exposed in comparison to the rest of the viral genome. Some restriction endonucleases can excise protein-free DNA fragments from the origin region of SV40 mini-chromosomes.[36] These studies showed that the protein-free region was about 400 bp long and from the "late transcribed" region which contains the SV40 large T antigen binding sites, tandem repeated sequences and promoters for late SV40 RNA synthesis. Staphylococcal nuclease was found to make single non-random cuts in the origin region and nearby "late" portion of SV40 mini-chromosomes.[37] However, even the origin region of the "super-compact" form of viral minichromosomes was found to be resistant to restriction endonucleases.[38] Prolonged formaldehyde treatment was found to crosslink histones to DNA except in a 325 bp stretch spanning the nuclease sensitive region.[39]

The nuclease digestion findings were supported by several studies using electron microscopy to examine the structure of SV40 minichromosomes. Saragosti and coworkers found that 15-25% of the viral minichromosomes had nucleosome free regions of about 249 bp and a maximum length of 385 bp.[40] Minichromosomes had 24 nucleosomes whether or not they had a nucleosome free region. The gap was found throughout the late phase of the virus cycle, and the gap was asymmetric with respect to the Bgl I cleavage site. Jakobovits and coworkers found the gap in 25% of the minichromosomes and placed it between 0.67 and 0.75 map units on the SV40 genome.[41]

The formation of a nucleosome free region is dependent upon specific DNA sequences. In two SV40 insertion mutants with the DNA fragment from 0.66-0.715 map units duplicated diametrically opposite to the original site in two alternative orientations, nucleosome free regions were seen at the sites of the duplications with the same frequency as at the original position.[42] In a host-substitution mutant in which the region spanning 0.67-0.73 map units was interspersed in four copies between cellular sequences, there was a nucleosome free region in 100% of the mini-chromosomes. When DNA insertions of variable size were located between the origin of DNA replication and the 21 bp repeats, the nuclease sensitive region was retained, but was moved to the late side of the inserts.[43] Viral replication was reduced in proportion to the size of the inserts and was independent of the DNA sequence of the insert. This suggests that the efficiency of the origin of replication is related to its proximity to the nucleosome free region. The 72- and 21-base pair repeats alone induced nuclease sensitive regions when transposed to other locations in the SV40 genome.[44] SV40 origin region deletion mutants have also been studied for formation of a nucleosome free region.[45] There was little or no effect if only one 21 bp repeat was present, but when both copies were disrupted, there was a pronounced reduction of the nuclease sensitive region of the minichromosome. There were no nuclease sensitive regions in minichromosomes with a TATA box and origin of replication but without the 21- and 72-bp repeats. On the basis of studies with deletion mutants, it was concluded that there were multiple DNA sequence determinants for formation of the nucleosome free region, but that none were completely independent of the others.

Restriction endonucleases were used to show that the origin specific nucleosome free region was present in nonencapsidated and partially encapsidated SV40 chromosomes, but not in virions.[46] Studies using radioactive psoralen analogs to selectively label the DNA of the nucleosome free region led to the conclusion that the region is not accessible to this reagent in minichromosomes from virions.[47] However, subsequent studies with this method suggested that the absence of a nucleosome free region in virion chromatin was an artifact of freezing and thawing protocols.[48] Studies with temperature sensitive mutants of the major capsid protein VP1 have provided good evidence that virion formation is associated with loss of the nucleosome free region.[49,50] SV40 tsC and tsB mutants are blocked at the initiation and propagation steps of virion assembly respectively at the restrictive temperature. At the restrictive temperature, minichromosomes from tsB mutants have an average nucleosome repeat length of 198 bp, similar to wild type SV40 minichromosomes. In contrast, minichromosomes from tsC mutants have a shorter average repeat length of 177 bp at the restrictive temperature. Remarkably, all of the tsC minichromosomes have nuclease hypersensitive regions at the restrictive temperature. The nucleosome free region appears to be established during viral DNA replication and lost during virion assembly.

SV40 large T antigen is the only detectable protein on the nucleosome free region.[51] In comparative studies of wild type SV40 and tsA58, a mutant with a large T antigen that is temperature sensitive for binding to site I, a nucleosome free promoter region was observed in a much larger proportion of minichromosomes from the mutant.[52] Thus, formation of the nucleosome region does not require large T antigen binding to site I, but this binding may determine the fraction of minichromosomes with nucleosome free regions. When HeLa cell nucleosomes were reconstituted onto SV40 DNA, a nucleosome free region was formed.[53] Topoisomerase II cleavage of SV40 DNA was higher in the nucleosome free region than in regions occupied by nucleosomes. Binding of topoisomerase II to the origin region also protected it from micrococcal nuclease digestion. There is reason to believe that the nucleosome free region is associated with transcription. All transcribed SV40 minichromosomes have a nucleosome free region.[54,55] However, nucleosome free regions alone may not be sufficient for transcription.[56] Superhelical stress may be involved in formation of the nucleosome free region. It is often thought that DNA in chromatin is not under superhelical stress. SV40 chromosomes can rapidly adjust their linking number in response to torsional stress caused by DNA intercalating drugs.[57-59] However, there is evidence that SV40 DNA in minichromosomes is under some superhelical stress.[60] The fact that the DNase I sensitive region in SV40 minichromosomes decreases as a function of X-ray dose,[61] suggests that superhelical stress may be involved in the formation or maintenance of the nucleosome free region.

Nuclease sensitive regions associated with transcribed regions and replication origins in mammalian cells[62-64] may be analogous to the nucleosome free regions of SV40 and polyomavirus. SV40 and polyomavirus have made many contributions to our understanding of chromatin structure, DNA replication and transcription as well as to our understanding of oncogenic transformation and cell cycle regulation. The focus of this book is the use of SV40 in understanding how anticancer drugs and DNA damaging agents disrupt DNA replication in mammalian cells.

REFERENCES

1. Hirt B. Selective extraction of polyoma DNA from infected mouse cell cultures. J Mol Biol 1967; 26:365-369.
2. Turler H, Beard P. Simian virus 40 and polyoma virus: growth, titration, transformation and purification of viral components. In: Mahy BWJ, ed. Virology, A Practical Approach. Oxford: IRL Press 1985:169-192.
3. Khoury G, Lai C-J. Preparation of simian virus 40 and its DNA. In: Jakoby WB, Pastan I, ed(s). Methods In Enzymology 58. Academic Press, Inc. 1979:404-412.
4. Pagano JS, Hutchison CA. Small, circular, viral DNA: preparation and analysis of SV40 and ϕX174 DNA. In: Maramorosch K, Koprowski H, ed(s). Methods in Virology 5. New York: Academic Press 1971:79-123.
5. Fendrick JL, Hallick L. Optimal conditions for titration of SV40 by the plaque assay method. J Virol Meth 1983; 7:93-102.
6. Rosenberg BH, Deutsch JF, Ungers GE. Growth and purification of SV40 virus for biochemical studies. J Virol Meth 1981; 3:167-176.
7. Tooze J. DNA tumor viruses. Cold Spring Harbor Laboratory 1991.
8. Fried M, Prives C. The biology of simian virus 40 and polyomavirus. In: Botchan M, Grodzicker T, Sharp PA, eds. Cancer Cells 4, DNA Tumor Viruses. Cold Spring Harbor Laboratory 1986; 4:1-16.
9. Challberg MD, Kelly TJ. Animal virus DNA replication. Annu Rev Biochem 1989; 58:671-717.
10. DePamphilis ML. Eukaryotic DNA replication: anatomy of an origin. Annu Rev Biochem 1993; 62:29-63.
11. DePamphilis ML, Chalifour LE, Carette MF, et al. Papovavirus chromosomes as a model for mammalian DNA replication. In: Cozzarelli N, ed. Mechanisms of DNA Replication and Recombination. New York: Alan R. Liss, Inc. 1983:423-447.
12. Meinke W, Hall MR, Goldstein DA. Proteins in intracellular simian virus 40 nucleoprotein complexes: comparison with simian virus 40 core proteins. J Virol 1975; 15:439-448.
13. Pett DM, Estes MK, Pagano JS. Structural proteins of simian virus 40. I. Histone characteristics of low-molecular-weight polypeptides. J Virol 1975; 15:379-385.
14. Lake RS, Barban S, Salzman NP. Resolutions and identification of the core deoxynucleoproteins of the simian virus 40. Biochem Biophys Res Commun 1973; 54:640-647.
15. Tan KB, Howe CC. Studies on viral DNA protein complexes isolated at different times after infection of monkey kidney cells with simian virus 40. Biochim Biophys Acta 1977; 478:99-108.

16. McMillen J, Consigli RA. Characterization of polyoma DNA-protein complexes. I. Electrophoretic identification of the proteins in a nucleoprotein complex isolated from polyoma-infected cells. J Virol 1974; 14:1326-1336.
17. Fey G, Hirt B. Fingerprints of polyoma virus proteins and mouse histones. Cold Spring Harbor Symp Quant Biol 1975; 39:235-241.
18. Griffith JD. Chromatin structure deduced from a minichromosome. Science 1975; 187:1202.
19. Germond JE, Hirt B, Oudet P et al. Folding of the DNA double helix in chromatin-like structures from simian virus 40. Proc Natl Acad Sci USA 1975; 72:1843-1847.
20. Schaffhausen BS, Benjamin TL. Deficiency in histone acetylation in nontransforming host range mutants of polyoma virus. Proc Natl Acad Sci USA 1976; 73:1092-1096.
21. Puerta C, Hernández F, López-Alarcón L et al. Acetylation of histone H2A.H2B dimers facilitates transcription. Biochem Biophys Res Commun 1995; 210:409-416.
22. Bates AD, Maxwell A, Rickwood D ed. DNA topology. Oxford: IRL Press 1993.
23. Varshavsky AJ, Bakayev VV, Chumakov PM et al. Minichromosomes of simian virus 40: presence of histone H1. Nucleic Acids Res 1976; 3:2101-2113.
24. Bellard M, Oudet P, Germond JE et al. Subunit structure of simian-virus-40 minichromosome. Eur J Biochem 1976; 70:543-553.
25. Varshavsky AJ, Nedospasov SA, Shmatchenko VV et al. Compact form of SV40 viral minichromosome is resistant to nuclease: possible implications for chromosome structure. Nucleic Acids Res 1977; 4:3303-3325.
26. Muller U, Zentgraf H, Eicken I et al. Higher order structure of simian virus 40 chromatin. Science 1978; 201:406-415.
27. Zentgraf H, Keller W, Muller U. The structure of SV40 chromatin. Philos Trans R Soc London 1978; B283:299-303.
28. Keller W, Muller U, Eicken I et al. Biochemical and ultrastructural analysis of SV40 chromatin. Cold Spring Harbor Symp Quant Biol 1978; 42:227-244.
29. Chen YH, MacGregor JP, Goldstein DA et al. Histone modifications in simian virus 40 and in nucleoprotein complexes containing supercoiled viral DNA. J Virol 1979; 30:218-224.
30. La Bella F, Romani M, Vesco C et al. High mobility group proteins 1 and 2 are present in simian virus 40 provirions, but not virions. Nucleic Acids Res 1981; 9:121-131.
31. Jeong S, Lauderdale JD, Stein A. Chromatin assembly on plasmid DNA in vitro. Apparent spreading of nucleosome alignment from one region of pBR327 by histone H5. J Mol Biol 1991; 222:1131-1147.

32. Halmer L, Gruss C. Influence of histone H1 on the in vitro replication of DNA and chromatin. Nucleic Acids Res 1995; 23: 773-778.

33. Nedospasov SA, Bakayev VV, Georgiev GP. Chromosome of the mature virion of simian virus 40 contains H1 histone. Nucleic Acids Res 1978; 5:2847-2860.

34. Varshavsky AJ, Sundin OH, Bohn MJ. SV40 viral minichromosome: preferential exposure of the origin of replication as probed by restriction endonucleases. Nucleic Acids Res 1978; 5:3469-3477.

35. Scott WA, Wigmore DJ. Sites in simian virus 40 chromatin which are preferentially cleaved by endonucleases. Cell 1978; 15: 1511-1518.

36. Varshavsky AJ, Sundin OH, Bohn M. A stretch of "late" SV40 viral DNA about 400 bp long which includes the origin of replication is specifically exposed in SV40 minichromosomes. Cell 1979; 16:453-466.

37. Sundin O, Varshavsky A. Staphylococcal nuclease makes a single non-random cut in the simian virus 40 viral minichromosome. J Mol Biol 1979; 132:535-546.

38. Das GC, Allison DP, Niyogi SK. Sites including those of origin and termination of replication are not freely available to single-cut restriction endonucleases in the supercompact form of simian virus 40 minichromosome. Biochem Biophys Res Commun 1979; 89:17-25.

39. Solomon MJ, Varshavsky A. Formaldehyde-mediated DNA-protein crosslinking: a probe for in vivo chromatin structures. Proc Natl Acad Sci USA 1985; 82:6470-6474.

40. Saragosti S, Moyne G, Yaniv M. Absence of nucleosomes in a fraction of SV40 chromatin between the origin of replication and the region coding for the late leader RNA. Cell 1980; 20:65-73.

41. Jakobovits EB, Bratosin S, Aloni Y. A nucleosome-free region in SV40 minichromosomes. Nature 1980; 285:263-265.

42. Jakobovits EB, Bratosin S, Aloni Y. Formation of a nucleosome-free region in SV40 minichromosomes is dependent upon a restricted segment of DNA. Virol 1982; 120:340-348.

43. Innis JW, Scott WA. DNA replication and chromatin structure of simian virus 40 insertion mutants. Mol Cell Biol 1984; 4: 1499-1507.

44. Jongstra J, Reudelhuber TL, Oudet P et al. Introduction of altered chromatin structures by simian virus 40 enhancer and promoter elements. Nature 1984; 307:708-714.

45. Gerard RD, Montelone BA, Walter CF et al. Role of specific simian virus 40 sequences in the nuclease-sensitive structure in viral chromatin. Mol Cell Biol 1985; 5:52-58.

46. Milavetz B. Analysis of the origin-specific nucleosome-free region of SV40 encapsidation intermediates. Virol 1986; 153:310-313.

47. Kondoleon SK, Robinson GW, Hallick LM. SV40 virus particles lack a psoralen-accessible origin and contain an altered nucleoprotein structure. Virol 1983; 129:261-273.

48. Kondoleon SK, Kurkinen NA, Hallick LM. The SV40 nucleosome-free region is detected throughout the virus life cycle. Virol 1989; 173:129-135.

49. Blasquez V, Stein A, Ambrose C et al. Simian virus 40 protein VP1 is involved in spacing nucleosomes in minichromosomes. J Mol Biol 1986; 191:97-106.

50. Ambrose C, Blasquez V, Bina M. A block in initiation of simian virus 40 assembly results in the accumulation of minichromosomes containing an exposed regulatory region. Proc Natl Acad Sci USA 1986; 83:3287-3291.

51. Weiss E, Ghose D, Schultz P et al. T-antigen is the only detectable protein on the nucleosome-free origin region of isolated simian virus 40 minichromosomes. Chromosoma 1985; 92:391-400.

52. Kube D, Milavetz B. Generation of a nucleosome-free promoter region in SV40 does not require T-antigen binding to site I. Virol 1989; 172:100-105.

53. Capranico G, Jaxel C, Roberge M et al. Nucleosome positioning as a critical determinant for the DNA cleavage sites of mammalian DNA topoisomerase II in reconstituted simian virus 40 chromatin. Nucleic Acids Res 1990; 18:4553-4559.

54. Weiss E, Ruhlmann C, Oudet P. Transcriptionally active SV40 minichromosomes are restriction enzyme sensitive and contain a nucleosome-free origin region. Nucleic Acids Res 1986; 14:2045-2058.

55. Choder M, Bratosin S, Aloni Y. A direct analysis of transcribed minichromosomes: all transcribed SV40 minichromosomes have a nuclease-hypersensitive region within a nucleosome free domain. EMBO J 1984; 3:2929-2936.

56. Lee M-S, Garrard WT. Uncoupling gene activity from chromatin structure: Promoter mutations can inactivate transcription of the yeast *HSP82* gene without eliminating nucleosome-free regions. Proc Natl Acad Sci USA 1992; 89:9166-9170.

57. Snapka RM, Permana PA. SV40 DNA replication intermediates: analysis of drugs which target mammalian DNA replication. BioEssays 1993; 15:121-127.

58. Esposito F, Sinden RR. Supercoiling in prokaryotic and eukaryotic DNA: changes in response to topological perturbation of plasmids in *E. coli* and SV40 in vitro, in nuclei and in CV-1 cells. Nucleic

Acids Res 1987; 15:5105-5124.

59. Chu Y, Hsu M-T. Ellipticine increases the superhelical density of intracellular SV40 DNA by intercalation. Nucleic Acids Res 1992; 20:4033-4038.

60. Barsoum J, Berg P. Simian virus 40 minichromosomes contain torsionally strained DNA molecules. Mol Cell Biol 1985; 5:3048-3057.

61. Bakayev VV, Yugai AA, Luchnik AN. Effect of X-ray induced DNA damage on DNase I hypersensitivity of SV40 chromatin: relation to elastic torsional strain in DNA. Nucleic Acids Res 1985; 13:7079-7093.

62. Grunstein M. Histones as regulators of genes. Sci Am 1992; 267:68-74B.

63. Reitman M, Felsenfeld G. Developmental regulation of topoisomerase II sites and DNase I-hypersensitive sites in the chicken β-globin locus. Mol Cell Biol 1990; 10:2774-2786.

64. Berberich S, Leffak M. DNase-sensitive chromatin structure near a chromosomal origin of bidirectional replication of the avian α-globin locus. DNA Cell Biol 1993; 12:703-714.

CHAPTER 2

ANALYSIS OF SV40 DNA REPLICATION INTERMEDIATES

Robert M. Snapka

Experimental methods used to analyze DNA replication in mammalian or microbial chromosomes are especially powerful when applied to SV40 because of its small size, circularity, selective extractability and known DNA sequence. The most important methods used in the study of SV40 DNA replication are described below with references to studies making use of them.

EXTRACTION OF VIRAL DNA AND CHROMATIN

The Hirt lysis was originally developed for selective extraction of polyoma virus DNA from infected mouse cells,[1] but it works just as well for SV40 or any other viral DNA of similar size. The extraction separates viral DNA from cellular chromosomes and most of the mitochondrial DNA. The basis of the procedure is high salt precipitation of the detergent sodium dodecyl sulfate (SDS) as it is complexed to chromatin. Under the extraction conditions, chromosomal proteins remain attached to DNA, and SDS is bound to the chromosomal proteins. Centrifugation causes the cellular chromosomes to form sticky pellets (the Hirt precipitate) and leaves most of the low molecular weight viral minichromosomes in the supernatant. The viral DNA in the Hirt extract supernatant remains bound to chromosomal proteins, and additional deproteinization by protease digestion and solvent extraction is required

The SV40 Replicon Model for Analysis of Anticancer Drugs,
edited by Robert M. Snapka. ©1996 R.G. Landes Company.

to obtain protein-free viral DNA. There is no selective retention of monomeric viral DNA in the cellular chromosomal pellet. The fraction of viral DNA in the pellet is a simple function of the pellet volume. This is not true for the minor class of oligomeric SV40 DNAs known as "circular oligomers" or "head-to-tail" dimers (chapter 8). The efficiency of the extraction is related to the size of the DNA and is decreased for larger DNAs. Covalent attachment of proteins to SV40 DNA does not decrease the efficiency of extraction. Contamination by mitochondrial DNA can be greatly reduced by adding Hirt lysing solution to a nuclear pellet obtained by centrifugation of a hypotonic cells' lysate.

Viral chromatin (minichromosomes) may also be selectively extracted from partially purified nuclei.[2-4] The viral minichromosomes tend to bind to the walls of pipets and centrifuge tubes, so it is advisable to quantitate the total labeled viral DNA before and after each minichromosome purification step. More than 95% of extracted viral chromatin can be lost by binding to the walls of pipets, centrifuge tubes and fraction tubes during a sucrose gradient purification.[5] In this case, the purified viral minichromosomes may be separated from many other cellular proteins, but they will represent only a small subset of the viral chromatin that may not be representative of the original population of minichromosomes.

RADIOLABELING OF SV40 DNA

Radioactive labeling of SV40 DNA for various purposes has been reviewed.[6,7] Agarose gel analysis of pulse-labeled viral replication intermediates requires high specific activity tritiated thymidine (250 µCi/ml, 70 Ci/mmol). The viral DNA is quickly extracted and processed for electrophoresis to minimize radiolytic nicking. When the effects of drugs or DNA-damaging treatments on SV40 DNA replication intermediates are being studied, untreated controls are crucial in order to detect DNA nicking from the added compounds. Radiolytic nicking of DNA can be used as a tool in two-dimensional electrophoresis.[8] In this approach, the gel is sealed in plastic wrap and stored in the cold after the first dimension electrophoresis. After several days or weeks to allow radiolytic nicking, a second dimension gel electrophoresis is done.

Under non-denaturing conditions, additional radiolytic nicks will not affect forms with double and single strand breaks, but new spots or bands will arise due to the nicking of covalently closed forms. This approach was also used with high-resolution one-dimensional gel electrophoresis by dividing a sample into several aliquots that were analyzed after different times.[8] Replication intermediates can be distinguished from completely replicated forms by comparing patterns of pulse-labeled intermediates to patterns resulting from pulse-chase labeling protocols. Replication intermediates are selectively labeled by labeling times of five minutes or less.[9] Longer labeling times result in a progressively larger fraction of the label in completely replicated forms. A 15 min labeling saturates the replication intermediates without excessive label in completed forms. To "chase" label from replication intermediates into completely replicated forms, the labeling medium is removed, and the cells are washed 3-4 times (15 min per wash) with medium containing unlabeled thymidine (1.0-5.0 μM). Each new wash with chase medium improves the chase, but it is never complete. There is always some trace of replication intermediates, but in the best chase experiments these can only be detected with very long fluorographic exposures.

SUCROSE DENSITY GRADIENT ULTRACENTRIFUGATION

Sucrose density gradient ultracentrifugation has historically been the workhorse of SV40 and polyomavirus DNA replication studies, and it may still have advantages under certain circumstances. For the major SV40 intermediates, the sedimentation coefficients are: form I (superhelical SV40 DNA circles), 21S; form II (relaxed circles),16S; form III (double strand linear DNA),12-14S; intermediate Cairns structures (replicating circular DNAs with growing replication bubbles), 25S.[9] Alkaline sucrose gradients have been used to separate single stranded DNAs derived from denaturation of viral replication intermediates. Under alkaline conditions, full SV40 genome-length linear single strand DNA has a sedimentation coefficient of 16S, and single strand SV40 circular DNA has a sedimentation coefficient of 18S. Alkaline denaturation of form I DNA gives a very compact form with a high sedimentation coefficient.[10] Thus, alkaline sucrose gradients can be used to obtain good separation of form I SV40 DNA from other replication intermediates.[9] Sucrose gradient ultracentrifugation has often been used in combination with other methods like isopycnic ultracentrifugation (below) or purification of replication intermediates by chromatography on benzoylated naphthoylated DEAE-cellulose.[9,11] Although much of our basic knowledge of papovavirus DNA replication was obtained from studies making extensive use of sucrose gradients, the resolution is very poor even for the major replication intermediates. The electrophoretic gel techniques discussed below not only achieve wide, clean separations of the major forms, but can resolve intermediates differing only by a single supercoil or a single change in catenation linking number.

ISOPYCNIC CENTRIFUGATION

Superhelical DNA takes up less of an intercalating dye than does DNA with strand breaks. This differential uptake of dyes like ethidium bromide or propidium diiodide causes relaxed DNAs to have reduced buoyant density relative to superhelical forms in the presence of saturating amounts of the dyes. Isopycnic centrifugation in cesium chloride-propidium diiodide was used to separate the A-, B- and C-families of catenated dimers and demonstrated that the A-family dimers banded with relaxed forms, the C-family banded with superhelical DNA, and the B-family had an intermediate density consistent with being half relaxed and half superhelical.[8] This method can also separate intermediate Cairns structures according to their extent of replication, since the superhelical unreplicated portion becomes smaller as replication of the circular genome progresses.[12,13] The intermediate Cairns structures are distributed between the form I and form II bands in ethidium bromide-cesium chloride gradients, with the least replicated forms being near form I and the most extensively replicated being near the form II band. Isopycnic banding can also be used to separate single stranded and double stranded DNAs or to separate density labeled replication intermediates from unlabeled intermediates.[14] It is routinely used to separate viral DNA from other macromolecules such as RNA or proteins.

HIGH-RESOLUTION ELECTROPHORESIS

Gel electrophoresis can achieve very fine resolution of viral DNA replication intermediates which have small differences in size, shape or topology. Superhelical molecules can be resolved into separate bands, each of which represents a specific level of superhelicity, and catenated circles can be resolved on the basis of catenation linking number (below). Electrophoresis can be done under a wide variety of conditions to achieve resolutions of particular forms, and the different types of electrophoretic separations can be combined in two-dimensional gel electrophoresis. The high resolving power of electrophoresis, the sensitivity of fluorography, and the ability to specifically radiolabel replicating DNA to high specific activities combine to give a technology which can be used to detect and analyze even very minor DNA replication intermediates.

The experimental details of high-resolution electrophoretic methods have been described, and their use in studies of SV40 DNA replication have been reviewed.[15,16] The descriptions below are crucial for understanding the discussion in subsequent chapters.

ONE-DIMENSIONAL NEUTRAL AGAROSE GEL ELECTROPHORESIS

Agarose gel electrophoresis at neutral pH separates SV40 DNA replication intermediates by size and compactness.[15,17] The completely replicated forms of the viral genome are widely separated from one another, and the viral replication intermediates are separated from one another as a function of their degree of completion. Agarose gel electrophoresis at neutral pH can be exquisitely sensitive to small changes in structure or compactness.

Figure 2.1 is a diagram of a typical one-dimensional agarose gel pattern of pulse-labeled SV40 DNA replication intermediates. The pulse-labeled intermediates are visualized by tritium fluorography on X-ray film.[18] Three of the most prominent bands represent SV40 genomes that have completed replication during the pulse-labeling. Form I DNA is the covalently closed, superhelical viral genome. As a small superhelical DNA circle, it is the smallest and most compact normal viral intermediate and has the highest electrophoretic mobility. The superhelical turns in form I DNA are due to nucleosome structure before deproteinization (see

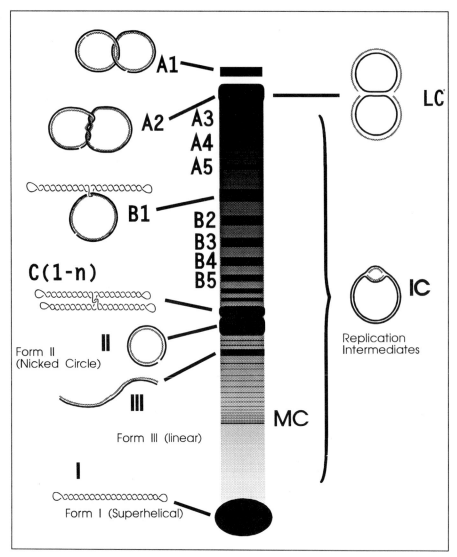

Fig. 2.1. Pattern of pulse-labeled SV40 DNA replication intermediates; separated by one-dimensional neutral agarose gel electrophoresis. I, form I (superhelical DNA circle) SV40 genome; II, form II (relaxed DNA circle); III, form III (double strand linear DNA); IC, intermediate Cairns replication forms; LC, late Cairns structure (terminus region unreplicated), A1-A5, relaxed-relaxed catenated SV40 daughter chromosomes with catenation linking numbers from 1 to 5; B1-B5, relaxed-superhelical catenated SV40 daughter chromosomes with catenation linking numbers 1-5; C(1-n), superhelical-superhelical catenated SV40 daughter chromosomes with catenation linking numbers from 1-several; MC, point where B-family catenated daughter chromosomes are no longer resolved from one another on one dimensional gels. Newly synthesized (and thus pulse-labeled) daughter DNA strands are indicated by light coloring and parental DNA strands by solid coloring in relaxed intermediates. Highly catenated SV40 daughter chromosomes are not normal DNA replication intermediates; they are seen only under conditions causing inhibition of topoisomerase II (hypertonic shock or presence of topoisomerase II inhibitors). The best resolution is obtained with 0.8% agarose submarine gels run at low voltage (0.8-1.0 V/cm) in TAE buffer (80 mM Tris HCl, pH 7.5, 5 mM sodium acetate, 1.0 mM sodium EDTA).

chapter 1). A single-strand DNA break or "nick" converts form I DNA to form II (relaxed circular) DNA. The relaxed DNA circle has the same mass or size (in base pairs) as form I, but it is much less compact. The decrease in compactness makes it more resistant to sieving through the pores of the gel matrix, thus, its electrophoretic mobility is greatly reduced. The form II molecules make a band well behind the form I band on agarose gels. Although form II DNA may be nicked, it can also be relaxed but covalently closed. The covalently closed, relaxed DNA circles co-migrate with the nicked circles in a neutral first dimensional gel, but they can be separated easily in the second dimension electrophoresis (for instance, the chloroquine second dimension described below). A double strand DNA break converts form I DNA to form III (double strand linear) DNA. The form III DNA is also much less compact than form I and has reduced electrophoretic mobility. However, it has a higher electrophoretic mobility than form II because it is able to "snake" or "reptate" through the pores of the gel matrix. Thus, the band of form III viral DNA is located just ahead of the form II band, but well behind the form I band on a neutral one-dimensional agarose gel pattern of SV40 replication intermediates (Fig. 2.1).

As DNA replication is initiated on an SV40 chromosome, a replication "eye" or "bubble" is formed at the origin of replication. The replication bubble grows in size as the replication forks move away from one another and eventually meet at the viral terminus of DNA replication, 180° from the origin or replication. The "theta-form" replication intermediates are covalently closed and retain the nucleosomal chromatin structure so that they are superhelical after deproteinization. By the time the replication forks meet at the terminus region, the replication intermediate has doubled in size. It is also relaxed since there is very little unreplicated region remaining, and the daughter chromosomes are gapped. The increase in size and the decrease in compactness throughout replication cause the replication intermediates to have progressively reduced electrophoretic mobility. In a one-dimensional neutral agarose gel pattern, these theta-form replication intermediates, also known as intermediate Cairns structures, form a continuous smear extending from the form I band to a point well behind the form

II band (Fig. 2.1). At this point the late Cairns structure is about 95% replicated and appears as a "figure eight" in electron micrographs. The smear of intermediate Cairns structures becomes denser as the extent of replication increases, and the late Cairns structures themselves are seen on fluorograms as a very dense band. This is because the rate of DNA replication slows progressively as more of the SV40 chromosome is replicated. There is a pause at the point of the late Cairns structures.[9,19] This slowing is probably due to changes in utilization of topoisomerases (chapter 4).

Replication is often completed without complete reduction of parental DNA strand linkage. This results in catenated daughter chromosomes (or catenated SV40 dimers) which are linked once for every turn of the Watson-Crick double helix that was not removed during replication.[17] The two daughter chromosomes making up a catenated dimer may both be relaxed (an A-family dimer), or one may be relaxed and one superhelical (a B-family dimer), or both may be superhelical (a C-family dimer).[17] The fully relaxed A-family catenated dimers are the least compact, and the fully superhelical C-family dimers are the most compact. The relaxed-superhelical B-family dimers have an intermediate compactness. This means that the compact C-family dimers tend to have the highest electrophoretic mobility, whereas the A-family catenated dimers have the lowest mobility. However, the separation of catenated dimers is complicated by the fact that their compactness and electrophoretic mobility also tend to increase with increasing catenation linking number. Each increase in catenation linking number causes a discrete increase in compactness and in electrophoretic mobility. Thus, the A- and B-family catenated dimer families form overlapping ladders of bands in one-dimensional neutral agarose gel electrophoretic patterns (Fig. 2.1). The level of catenation in each band can be determined by band counting from the known positions of the A1 and B1 dimer bands. The C-family dimers with low levels of catenation are not resolved from one another on the one dimensional gel. Normally, catenated A- and B-family SV40 daughter chromosomes with linking numbers of 1-3 can be observed, but inhibition of topoisomerase II can cause catenation linking numbers of over 25 (chapter 4).

The standard one dimensional neutral agarose gel electrophoresis gives much higher resolution and proportionally more information than sucrose gradient ultracentrifugation. However, even greater resolution is achieved with two-dimensional gel electrophoresis techniques. Neutral agarose gel electrophoresis is used routinely as the first dimension separation for various two-dimensional gels. This standardization greatly simplifies the identification of new aberrant replication intermediates in second dimension gel patterns.

TWO-DIMENSIONAL AGAROSE GEL ELECTROPHORESIS

Although one-dimensional gel electrophoresis can achieve very high resolution of viral replication intermediates, much higher resolution can be achieved by two-dimensional gel electrophoresis in which the second dimension electrophoresis is done under very different conditions at a right angle to the first. The changes in the second dimension electrophoresis can involve altered buffer composition (such as pH or ionic strength), gel porosity, electric field protocol or the presence of DNA-binding dyes. The second dimension can also be identical to the first, but following some treatment of the first dimension gel lane such as irradiation or in-gel digestion with a nuclease. Since the basis of each separation is understood, the two-dimensional gel represents a logic system which can be used to deduce the nature of unknown aberrant viral replication intermediates. For two dimensional gels, the first dimension gel lane can either be cut out and placed in a second-dimension gel or the entire gel can be saturated with a new electrophoresis buffer before electrophoresis at a right angle to the first dimension. When the first dimension gel lane is cut out, it can either be placed in a slot in the second dimension gel or the second dimension gel can be cast around it. The routine use of neutral agarose gel electrophoresis as a standard first dimension is advisable since the relative positions of the major intermediates is well established for those conditions and the basis of separation is well understood.

Neutral-neutral two-dimensional gel electrophoresis

Two dimensional gels in which both dimensions are run in the same buffer can yield additional information if the porosity of the gel is changed for the second dimension. This method was first used to show that the A- and B-family ladders of catenated dimer bands represented two different groups and to separate them from the intermediate Cairns structures and the late Cairns structure.[8]

Neutral-alkaline two-dimensional gel electrophoresis

In two-dimensional neutral-alkaline gels, the first dimension is run under conditions of neutral pH, and the gel lane is excised from the gel. The excised first dimension gel lane is then soaked in alkaline buffer and imbedded in a second-dimension gel cast in the same alkaline buffer.[8,15] The alkaline buffer denatures the viral replication intermediates, separating the DNA strands. Only the daughter, or nascent, DNA strands have the tritiated thymidine pulse label, so parental strands do not contribute to the fluorographic image. The parental strands can influence the pattern when they remain either covalently or topologically attached to the labeled daughter strands. The form I band from the first dimension gel gives rise to a single spot in the alkaline second dimension since it is covalently closed, and the labeled daughter DNA strand cannot separate from the unlabeled parental strand (Fig. 2.2). The form III band from the first dimension also gives rise to a single spot in the alkaline second dimension since it denatures into full genome-length single strand DNA. The unlabeled parental strands co-migrate with the labeled nascent strands in the second dimension but do not contribute to the fluorographic image. The first dimension form II band gives rise to two spots in the alkaline second dimension. One corresponds to single strand linear DNA, arising from form II molecules in which the nick is in the nascent strand, and the other corresponds to single strand DNA circles from form II molecules in which the nick is in the parental strand. Although form I DNA is converted to form II by a single strand DNA break and to form III by a double strand DNA break, additional single strand breaks do not alter the electrophoretic behavior of forms II and III under non-denaturing conditions. If additional DNA strand breaks are present, they are evident in second dimension alkaline gels where they produce a "tail" of subgenomic labeled fragments extending from the form II and III spots in the

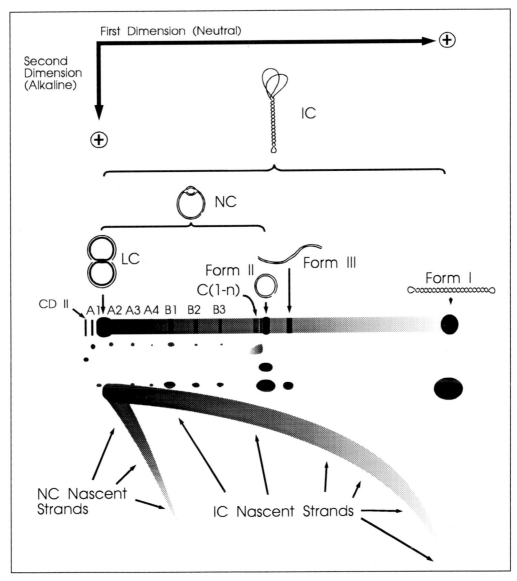

Fig. 2.2. Two-dimensional neutral-alkaline gel separation of pulse-labeled normal SV40 DNA replication intermediates. NC, nicked Cairns structures; CD II, circular (head-to-tail) dimers. Other abbreviations are the same as in Figure 2.1. The second dimension gel is 1.5% agarose in alkaline buffer (30 mM NaOH, 2.0 mM EDTA, 1.0 mM EGTA). It is also a submarine gel and is run at 2.33 V/cm.

direction of the second dimension electrophoresis. By definition, form I has no DNA strand breaks. When a pronounced tail of subgenomic fragments is seen to extend from the form I spot in an alkaline second dimension, it is evidence of alkaline-sensitive sites, such as abasic sites. The DNA strand breaks are produced at these alkaline-sensitive sites in the form I DNA by the alkaline conditions of the second dimension buffer.

Nascent DNA strands from growing replication bubbles range in size from a few nucleotides, arising from the small replication bubbles of the earliest replication intermediates, to full length linear strands from late Cairns structures. These nascent strands thus give rise to an arc in the alkaline second dimension gel. This arc runs from the position of the form I band to the position of the late Cairns band in the first dimension and from the dye front to the level of full length linear single strands (marked by the form III spot) in the alkaline second dimension (Fig. 2.2). The arc is asymptotic to a line running through the form I spot perpendicular to the direction of the first dimension electrophoresis. Form I DNA can be considered the starting point of the Cairns replication intermediates—zero percent replicated. Arcs in two-dimensional gel patterns are indications of families of normal or abnormal replication intermediates. By observing which completed form the arc approaches asymptotically, the investigator can obtain a clue to the nature of an arc of abnormal intermediates produced by a drug exposure. A smaller second arc is seen in a two-dimensional neutral-alkaline gel pattern of normal SV40 intermediates. This arc is composed of nascent strands from nicked Cairns structures. Normal, superhelical intermediate Cairns structures are distributed between the form I band and the late Cairns structure band in the first dimension, but nicked Cairns structures are distributed between the form II band and the late Cairns structure. As shown in Figure 2.2, the arc from nicked Cairns structures is asymptotic to the form II band in the two-dimensional pattern. The form II nicked circle, then, is the "zero percent replicated" starting form for this family of replication intermediates. The relaxed circular (head-to-tail) dimer is also indicated. This is a double-sized SV40 DNA circle which is generated by rare recombinational events. These recombinational events may occur at moving replication forks.[20]

Neutral-chloroquine two-dimensional gel electrophoresis

In neutral-chloroquine gels, the first dimension buffer is replaced with a buffer containing the strong DNA intercalating and unwinding drug chloroquine.[15] Intercalators unwind negative superhelical DNA so that it is no longer supercoiled. At the same time, they will overwind covalently closed, relaxed DNA circles, causing positive supercoils. The effect is a reversal of compactness for covalently closed DNA circles. Negatively supercoiled form I DNA is very compact and fast migrating in neutral first dimension gels lacking chloroquine, but chloroquine in the second dimension gel titrates out the negative supercoils converting form I to a "relaxed circle" which is much less compact. Covalently closed, relaxed circles (form II, but not nicked) become positively supercoiled and much more compact in chloroquine. Since the catenated dimer families differ from one another by the superhelicity of the daughter chromosomes making up each dimer, the three families behave differently in chloroquine. Chloroquine will not alter the overall structure or topology of DNAs that are not covalently closed (linear DNA and nicked circular DNA). Thus, the A-family catenated dimer bands make a straight diagonal on a two-dimensional neutral-chloroquine gel (see chapters 4 and 8). The non-linear behavior of the B-family catenated dimer ladder in two-dimensional neutral-chloroquine gels has been interpreted as evidence that high levels of catenation decrease superhelicity in the daughter chromosomes making up each dimer.[21] A two-dimensional neutral-chloroquine gel separation of pulse-labeled normal SV40 DNA replication intermediates is shown in Figure 2.3.

Neutral-pulsed field two-dimensional gel electrophoresis

Remarkable separations can be achieved by using pulsed-field second dimension electrophoresis following a first dimension normal electrophoresis at constant voltage. The one problem with pulsed-field gels is that the electrophoretic behavior of unusual DNA structures is not always well understood. Thus, it may be difficult to deduce the structure of a new intermediate observed in a two-dimensional gel pattern involving pulsed-field electrophoresis.

Figure 2.4 shows a two-dimensional neutral-pulsed-field separation of highly catenated SV40 daughter chromosomes produced by exposure of infected cells to a strong topoisomerase II inhibitor.

The ladders of A- and B-family catenated dimer bands are well separated in the region in which they overlap in the first dimension. The A-family bands representing dimers of low catenation linking number are also well separated from the late Cairns replication intermediates. The ladders of A- and B-family catenated dimers cross four times, and the B-family dimer ladder shows a

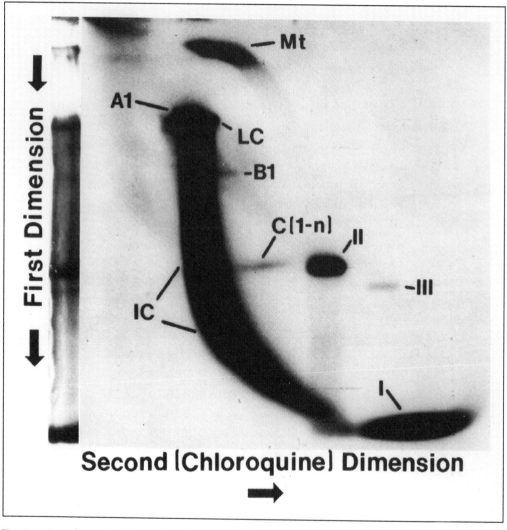

Fig. 2.3. Two-dimensional neutral-chloroquine gel electrophoresis of normal SV40 DNA replication intermediates. Abbreviations are the same as in Figures 2.1 and 2.2. Second dimension chloroquine gels are run at 2.4 V/cm for 10 h in TBE buffer (89 mM Tris base, 89 mM boric acid, 2 mM EDTA) containing 15 µg/ml chloroquine.

cusp at the point where individual bands can no longer be resolved (MC in the first dimension gel). The point at which
B-family dimers are no longer resolved from one another (MC) is
also the point at which they begin to overlap the diagonal line of
highly catenated A-family dimer bands in two-dimensional

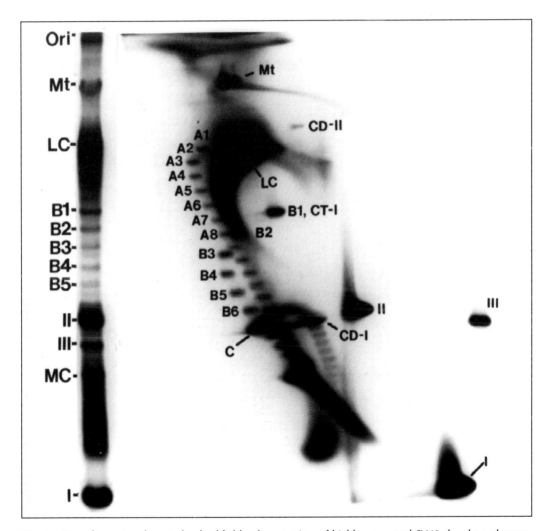

Fig. 2.4. *Two-dimensional neutral-pulsed-field gel separation of highly catenated SV40 daughter chromosomes. SV40-infected cells were exposed to 100 µg/ml A-74932, a topoisomerase II antagonist, during the
last 15 min of a 30 min pulse-labeling of replicating viral DNA with tritiated thymidine. A standard first
dimensional submarine agarose gel electrophoresis was done at 1.0 V/cm (36 hr). The first dimension gel lane
was excised with a scalpel and then cast directly in a second dimension gel (250 ml BioRad Fastlane agarose
in 0.25X Tris-Borate-EDTA buffer, 19.5 X 22.5 cm tray). The second dimension electrophoresis was done at
a right angle to the direction of the first dimension gel in a BioRad Chef DR II pulse unit (18 hr, 1.0 sec pulse,
175V). A-74932 was a gift from Abbott Laboratories.*

neutral-chloroquine gels (chapter 4). In those gels it has not been possible to separate the lower ends of the A- and B-family catenated dimer ladders (representing catenation linking numbers greater than 25). This is probably because the high level of catenation has prevented any superhelicity in the covalently closed member of each highly catenated B-dimer, and the B-family dimers without superhelicity would be difficult to distinguish from A-family dimers. The pulsed-field second dimension has achieved the difficult separation of the most highly catenated A- and B-family dimers. Conditions causing accumulation of highly catenated SV40 daughter chromosomes cause the band of unresolved C-family dimers to broaden backwards in one dimensional neutral gels. In this neutral-pulsed-field two-dimensional gel, it can be seen that the C-dimers first show a decrease in electrophoretic mobility, then begin to show increased electrophoretic mobility as they resolve into bands at higher levels of catenation. This behavior may be related to a loss of superhelicity in the daughter chromosomes with increasing catenation, similar to that suggested for the B-family dimers.[21] The basis for electrophoretic behavior in the pulsed-field dimension is not clear in many cases. For instance, the mobility in this dimension decreases with the first two increases in catenation (the A2 and A3 dimers), then progressively increases with increasing catenation. The same phenomenon is seen in the B-dimer ladder.

Neutral-denaturation-renaturation two-dimensional gel electrophoresis

Following a first dimension neutral gel electrophoresis, SV40 DNA replication intermediates can be denatured and renatured in the gel by equilibrating it first in alkaline and then in neutral pH buffers. The covalently closed forms renature, but the nascent strands are removed from replication intermediates. In chapter 8, this method is combined with a chloroquine second dimension to simplify a complex gel pattern and to demonstrate abnormal replication intermediates for the SV40 circular oligomers.

Neutral-nuclease-neutral two-dimensional gel electrophoresis

Following first dimension neutral electrophoresis, the gel lane can be excised and soaked in an enzyme reaction buffer. Once it is equilibrated in the reaction buffer, concentrated enzyme can be soaked into the gel. After a sufficient time, determined by trial and error, the reaction is stopped by soaking the gel lane in the original SDS-containing first dimension electrophoresis buffer. The gel lane is then imbedded in a new neutral agarose gel, and a second neutral gel electrophoresis is carried out at a 90 degree angle to the first. In this case, the first and second dimension electrophoretic conditions may be identical, but the structure of the replication intermediates is changed by the nuclease digestion. Between the first and second dimensions, restriction endonucleases can be used to introduce double strand DNA breaks at specific DNA sequences. S1 nuclease has also been used between the first and second dimensions to digest single stranded regions at replication forks (P. Permana, unpublished data).

Identification of intermediates making up bands, spots and arcs in agarose gel patterns

A wide variety of techniques can be applied to the assignment of specific DNA structures to the elements making up gel patterns. Many structures have been confirmed by electron microscopy, including the late and intermediate Cairns structures, the three families of catenated dimers and sigma forms with broken replication forks. These are reviewed in later chapters. As discussed in chapter 3, the structure of sigma forms and the identification of a smear of subgenomic linear fragments as detached replication bubbles was done by experiments with S1 nuclease which digests the single stranded regions at replication forks. A partial digest of normal SV40 replication intermediates with S1 nuclease produces random breaks at DNA replication forks. The resulting sigma and linear forms are similar to those produced by the topoisomerase I poison camptothecin (CPT). Completely replicated forms like forms I, II and III are selectively labeled in pulse-chase experiments, whereas short pulse-labeling selectively labels intermediates in the process of DNA synthesis. Controlled nicking of superhelical forms by radiolysis or DNase I gives the corresponding relaxed forms. This can be done either before the first dimension gel electrophoresis or "in the gel" between first and second dimension electrophoretic steps in a two dimensional gel. As discussed above, this technique has been used to demonstrate the relationship between the three catenated dimer families. Relaxation of superhelical forms can also be done with topoisomerase I which produces covalently closed relaxed forms.

Figure 2.5 shows a two-dimensional neutral-chloroquine gel separation of highly catenated dimers which were treated with topoisomerase I before the first dimension electrophoresis. The superhelical daughter chromosomes in B- and C-family catenated dimers were completely relaxed but remained covalently closed. Under the conditions of the first dimension neutral agarose gel electrophoresis, these dimers were indistinguishable from the corresponding A-family catenated dimers in which both daughter chromosomes are relaxed due to single strand DNA breaks. The relaxed B- and C-family dimers were separated from the A-family dimers and from one another in the chloroquine second dimension electrophoresis. Intercalation of chloroquine causes positive supercoiling in covalently closed relaxed DNA circles, increasing their compactness and electrophoretic mobility in the chloroquine second dimension electrophoresis. This experiment confirms the structures and relationships of the three catenated dimer families.

The structures of viral replication intermediates can also be confirmed by using other techniques to purify them or selectively remove them. Intermediates crosslinked to protein can be purified, or selectively removed, by filtration through glass fiber filters or nitrocellulose filters (discussed below). Superhelical or partially superhelical intermediates can be purified by isopycnic ultracentrifugation in the presence of intercalating dyes, and replication intermediates with single strand gaps can be purified on columns of benzoylated naphthoylated DEAE-cellulose (both techniques discussed above).

ELECTRON MICROSCOPY

Electron microscopy can be used in a number of ways to visualize SV40 DNA replication intermediates, both as DNA and as chromatin. Although the identities of viral replication intermediates giving rise to peaks in density gradient ultracentrifugation experiments and to bands in gel electrophoretic separations can

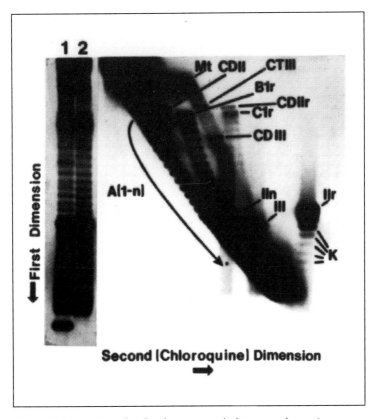

Fig. 2.5. Separation of A-family catenated dimers and topoisomerase I-relaxed B- and C-family catenated dimers by two-dimensional neutral-chloroquine gel electrophoresis. SV40-infected cells were pulse-labeled for 45 min with 40 μM proflavine present in the last 30 min. The DNA sample was divided into two aliquots; one served as a control without topoisomerase I relaxation, the other was relaxed with topoisomerase I (2 U/μg DNA) for 30 min at 37°C prior to gel electrophoresis. The two samples, labeled respectively "1" and "2," were electrophoresed in the first-dimension neutral buffer (top to bottom). A duplicate "2" lane was then equilibrated in chloroquine containing second dimension buffer. The second dimension chloroquine gel electrophoresis was carried out at a right angle to the first dimension neutral agarose gel electrophoresis (left to right). Abbreviations: K, Keller bands (relaxation intermediates of form I DNA); B1r, relaxed B-family catenated dimer with catenation linking number of one; C1r, relaxed C-family catenated dimer with catenation linking number of one; IIr, form II relaxed, IIn, form II nicked; CDIII, form III of the circular (head-to-tail) dimer; CDII, form II circular dimer nicked; CDIIr, form II circular dimer relaxed; A (1-n), A-family catenated dimers with linking numbers 1 to over 25; Mt, mitochondrial DNA; III, form III DNA. Relaxed B- and C-family catenated dimers with linking numbers higher than one make up the ladders beneath the B1r and C1r bands, with each successive band representing an increase of one in catenation linking number. Keller bands are covalently closed SV40 DNA circles with only a few superhelical turns.

usually be deduced on the basis of other considerations, electron microscopy has often been used to confirm these identifications. Many studies of viral DNA replication have been done largely or completely with electron microscopy. These same techniques are often used to study cellular chromosomes, but have been especially useful for the papovaviruses because of their small size, circular structure, ease of purification and known DNA sequences. The ability to cleave the SV40 genome at specific single-cut restriction endonuclease sites has greatly facilitated electron microscopy studies of asynchronous replication fork movement and use of secondary origins of replication.[22-24] This approach was also used to demonstrate that SV40 can terminate DNA replication at sequences other than the normal terminus region.[25] Unlike centrifugation and electrophoresis methods, electron microscopy alone cannot distinguish between parental DNA strands and daughter DNA strands, nor can it demonstrate covalent linkage of parental and daughter DNA strands. Potential artifacts of special concern for electron microscopy studies—in which the focus is often on minor fractions of viral replication intermediates—include contamination with cellular DNA, undetected overlays or contacts between normal intermediates, and re-annealing at DNA strand breaks such as broken replication forks. The ability of trimethylpsoralen to crosslink DNA duplexes at internucleosomal regions has been developed into a unique indirect method of studying chromatin structure in replicating SV40 genomes by electron microscopy.[26] Electron microscopy of viral chromatin itself is difficult since the nucleosome structure tends to obscure the path of the DNA helix and the overall structure of the genome.

FILTER ASSAYS

The small size and circular topology of the SV40 chromosome make it ideal for filter assays used to detect DNA damage such as protein-DNA crosslinks. Topoisomerase poisons such as camptothecin (a topoisomerase I poison) and teniposide (a topoisomerase II poison) stabilize DNA reaction intermediates in which the topoisomerase is covalently attached to the DNA at the site of a DNA strand break. These "cleavable complexes" or "protein-associated DNA strand breaks" can be quantitated by a rapid filter assay.[27] This assay can be done on the unprocessed Hirt lysate supernatant and gives a fraction of the pulse-labeled viral DNA that is crosslinked to protein. In 0.4 M guanidinium chloride, the glass fiber filters retain only those viral chromosomes crosslinked to protein, and in 4.0 M guanidinium chloride, all DNA is retained on the filter. Although histones are still noncovalently bound to the viral chromosomes in the Hirt extract supernatant, they are removed by the guanidinium chloride, a strong protein denaturant. The protein-crosslinked SV40 genomes bound to the filter in 0.4 M guanidinium chloride can be eluted and examined by high-resolution gel electrophoresis to determine if specific replication intermediates are selectively linked to the topoisomerase.[28] The K-SDS precipitation assay for topoisomerase-DNA complexes[29] can be adapted to SV40 to provide the same information. Circular DNAs can also be used as substrates for "nicked circle" assays for DNA damage.[5,30] In these assays, DNA containing lesions such as pyrimidine photodimers is treated with a damage-specific endonuclease that cleaves the DNA specifically at the lesions. Rapid denaturation-renaturation irreversibly denatures the nicked molecules, causing them to bind to nitrocellulose filters while the intact superhelical circles renature and pass through the filter. The ratio of filter-bound to total DNA can be used to calculate the average numbers of DNA lesions per DNA circle.

REFERENCES

1. Hirt B. Selective extraction of polyoma DNA from infected mouse cell cultures. J Mol Biol 1967; 26:365-369.
2. Oudet P, Weiss E, Regnier E. Preparation of simian virus 40 minichromosomes. In: Wassarman PM, Kornberg RD, eds. Nucleosomes. San Diego: Academic Press, Inc. 1989:14-25.
3. Griffith JD. Chromatin structure deduced from a minichromosome. Science 1975; 187:1202.
4. Bellard M, Oudet P, Germond JE et al. Subunit structure of simian-virus-40 minichromosome. Eur J Biochem 1976; 70:543-553.
5. Snapka RM, Linn SM. Efficiency of formation of pyrimidine dimers in SV40 chromatin in vitro. Biochemistry 1981; 20:68-72.
6. Pagano JS, Hutchison CA. Small, circular, viral DNA: preparation and analysis of SV40 and φX174 DNA. In: Maramorosch K, Koprowski H, eds. Methods in Virology 5. New York: Academic Press 1971:79-123.

7. Khoury G, Lai C-J. Preparation of simian virus 40 and its DNA. In: Jakoby WB, Pastan I, eds. Methods In Enzymology 58. San Diego: Academic Press, Inc. 1979:404-412.

8. Sundin O, Varshavsky A. Terminal stages of SV40 DNA replication proceed via multiply intertwined catenated dimers. Cell 1980; 21:103-114.

9. Levine AJ, Kang HY, Billheimer FE. DNA replication in SV40 infected cells, I. Analysis of replicating SV40 DNA. J Mol Biol 1970; 50:549-564.

10. Bauer W, Vinograd J. Circular DNA. In: Ts'o POP, ed. Basic Principles in Nucleic Acid Chemistry. New York: Academic Press, Inc. 1974:265-303.

11. Tapper DP, DePamphilis ML. Discontinuous DNA replication: accumulation of simian virus 40 DNA at specific stages in its replication. Mol Biol 1978; 120:401-422.

12. Jaenisch R, Mayer A, Levine AJ. Replicating SV40 molecules containing closed circular template DNA strands. Nature New Biology 1971; 233:72-75.

13. Sebring ED, Garon CF, Salzman NP. Superhelix density of replicating simian virus 40 DNA molecules. J Mol Biol 1974; 90:371-379.

14. Roman A, Dulbecco R. Fate of polyoma form I DNA during replication. J Virol 1975; 16:70-74.

15. Snapka RM, Permana PA, Marquit G et al. Two-dimensional agarose gel analysis of simian virus 40 DNA replication intermediates. Methods: a companion to methods in enzymology 1991; 3:73-82.

16. Snapka RM, Permana PA. SV40 DNA replication intermediates: analysis of drugs which target mammalian DNA replication. BioEssays 1993; 15:121-127.

17. Varshavsky A, Sundin O, Ozkaynak E et al. Final stages of DNA replication: multiply intertwined catenated dimers as SV40 segregation intermediates. In: Cozzarelli NR ed. Mechanisms of DNA Replication and Recombination. New York: Alan R. Liss 1983: 463-494.

18. Pulleyblank DE, Booth GM. Improved methods for the fluorographic detection of weak beta-emitting radioisotopes in agarose and acrylamide gel electrophoresis media. J Biomed Biophys Meth 1981; 4:339-346.

19. Levine AJ, Van der Vliet PC, Sussenbach JS. The replication of papovavirus and adenovirus DNA. Current Topics in Microbiol Immunol 1976; 73:67-124.

20. Snapka RM. Topoisomerase inhibitors can selectively interfere with different stages of simian virus 40 DNA replication. Mol Cell Biol 1986; 6:4221-4227.

21. Permana PA, Ferrer CA, Snapka RM. Inverse relationship between catenation and superhelicity in newly replicated simian virus 40 daughter chromosomes. Biochem Biophys Res Commun 1995; 201:1510-1517.

22. Robberson DL, Crawford LV, Syrett C et al. Unidirectional replication of a minority of polyoma virus and SV40 DNAs. J Gen Virol 1975; 26:59-69.

23. Martin RG, Setlow VP. The initiation of SV40 DNA synthesis is not unique to the replication origin. Cell 1980; 20:381-391.

24. Tack LC, Proctor GN. Two major replicating simian virus 40 chromosome classes. Synchronous replication fork movement is associated with bound large T antigen during elongation. J Biol Chem 1987; 262:6339-6349.

25. Lai C-J, Nathans D. Non-specific termination of simian virus 40 DNA replication. J Mol Biol 1975; 97:113-118.

26. Sogo JM, Stahl H, Koller T et al. Structure of replicating simian virus 40 minichromosomes. The replication fork, core histone segregation and terminal structures. J Mol Biol 1986; 189:189-204.

27. Shin C-G, Strayer JM, Wani MA et al. Rapid evaluation of topoisomerase inhibitors: caffeine inhibition of topoisomerases in vivo. Teratogen Carcinogen Mutagen 1990; 10:41-52.

28. Shin C-G, Snapka RM. Patterns of strongly protein-associated simian virus 40 DNA replication intermediates resulting from exposures to specific topoisomerase poisons. Biochemistry 1990; 29:10934-10939.

29. Trask DK, DiDonato JA, Muller MT. Rapid detection and isolation of covalent DNA/protein complexes: application to topoisomerase I and II. EMBO J 1984; 3:671-676.

30. Kühnlein U, Penhoet EE, Linn S. An altered apurinic DNA endonuclease activity in group A and group D xeroderma pigmentosum fibroblasts. Proc Natl Acad Sci USA 1976; 73:1169-1173.

CHAPTER 3

CATASTROPHIC FAILURE OF DNA REPLICATION FORKS: STRUCTURAL AND RECOMBINATIONAL PATHWAYS

Robert M. Snapka

Disruption of DNA replication fork movement causes rapid changes in the topology and structure of replicating SV40 genomes. Replication begins on covalently closed circular SV40 minichromosomes with approximately 20-24 nucleosomes. When the viral DNA is extracted and deproteinized, it is superhelical, with one negative superhelical turn for each nucleosome that was present in the minichromosome.[1-3] Replication of a circular DNA chromosome such as SV40 presents two related topological problems: the swivel problem and the termination problem. The termination problem refers to the necessity of reducing the parental DNA strand linkage to zero by the end of DNA replication so that the daughter chromosomes can separate. If it were possible to replicate the SV40 genome without reducing the linkage of the parental strands, the resulting daughter chromosomes would be topologically linked once for each turn of the parental DNA helix—over 500 times. Topologically linked or "catenated" daughter chromosomes exist as normal minor replication intermediates in both eukaryotes and

The SV40 Replicon Model for Analysis of Anticancer Drugs,
edited by Robert M. Snapka. ©1996 R.G. Landes Company.

prokaryotes, but their catenation linking numbers are normally much lower—on the order of 1-3. No catenated chromosomes with linking numbers in the hundreds have ever been reported, and it is doubtful that such molecules could exist. Some enzymatic activity must continually reduce the linkage of the parental DNA strands during DNA replication.

The second topological problem in DNA replication is the swivel problem. A replication bubble is opened by unwinding the parental DNA strands at the origin of replication. Since the bubble region is unwound, the linkage of the two parental strands must now be restricted to the unreplicated part of the chromosome. As the replication bubble expands, the unreplicated part of the chromosome quickly becomes overwound (positive superhelicity). This positive superhelical stress is a barrier to continued replication fork movement. An enzymatic activity is required to reduce the linkage of the parental DNA strands and remove the superhelical stress. This is known as the swivel problem since a "swivel" or "nicking-closing" enzyme capable of transiently introducing single strand DNA breaks in the unreplicated region could serve this function. The swivel and termination problems are related since a single swivel activity could potentially solve both problems, reducing parental strand linkage to remove superhelical stress ahead of moving replication forks and reducing the linkage to zero by the end of replication. Chapter 4 will review evidence that a single swivel activity is insufficient and that complete replication of SV40 chromosomes requires the sequential action of two very different swivel enzymes.

In theory, either a type I or a type II topoisomerase could serve as the swivel activity.[4] A type I topoisomerase can only do this by carrying out its single strand DNA passing reaction on the unreplicated region ahead of the replication forks (Fig. 3.1). A type II topoisomerase can serve as a replication swivel by carrying out its double strand passing reaction on either the unreplicated region or on the replicated region behind the replication forks (Fig. 3.2). This is possible since the parental DNA strands are continuous through the replication forks.

Assuming that a swivel activity (either topoisomerase I or topoisomerase II) reduces parental DNA strand linkage during replication, the parental strands in partially replicated circular DNA

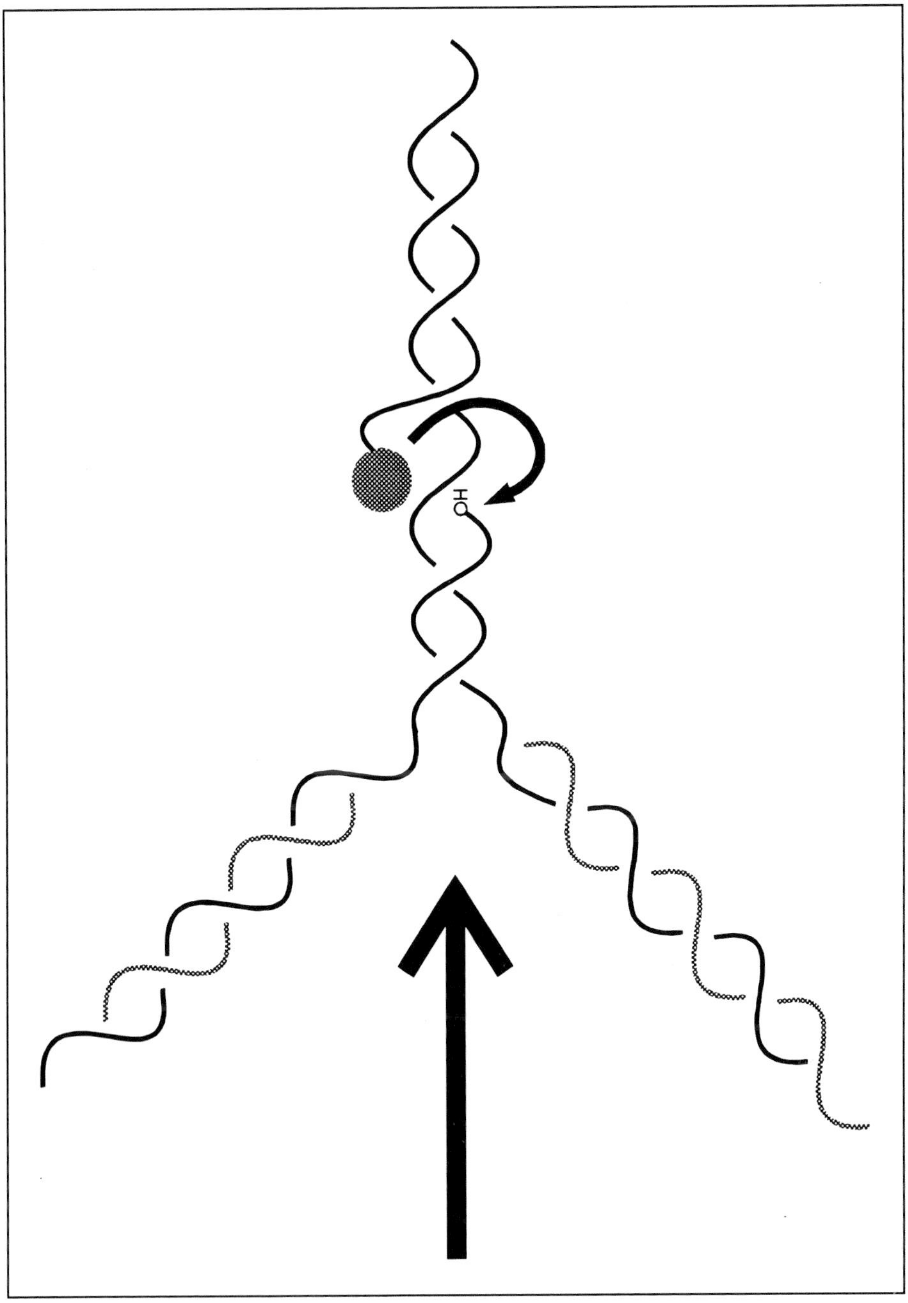

Fig. 3.1. Topoiso-merase I can act as a swivel for replica-tion fork movement by acting on the unreplicated region to reduce the link-age of parental DNA strands. Parental DNA strands are shown in black, and nascent daughter strands are shown in gray. Topoiso-merase I introduces a single strand DNA break in the double helix while becom-ing covalently at-tached to the DNA through a 3' phos-phoryl linkage. The other strand of the DNA helix is then passed through this single strand gap. Ligation to the free 5' hydroxyl group seals the gap and releases the enzyme.

Fig. 3.2. Topoisomerase II can serve as a swivel for DNA replication by carrying out its double strand passing reaction in the replicated region behind DNA replication forks. Topoisomerase II is composed of two identical subunits. It makes a double strand DNA break in which each subunit is covalently attached to the DNA through a 5' phosphoryl linkage. Another segment of DNA double helix is passed through the double strand gap. Ligation of the DNA strand break reverses the covalent bonds to the subunits. Since the parental DNA strands are continuous through the replication forks, this double strand passing reaction in the replicated region can reduce the linkage of the parental DNA strands in the molecule as a whole.

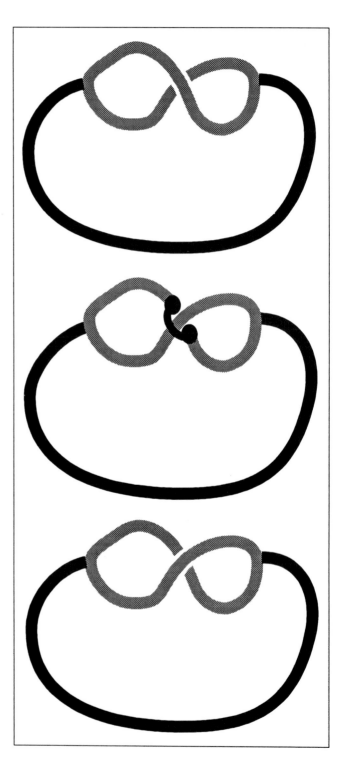

molecules will still have significant linkage and will be capable of having a linkage deficit after deproteinization. Partially completed SV40 replication intermediates are covalently closed and superhelical.[5-7] In one-dimensional neutral agarose gel electrophoresis, the normal superhelical Cairns structures are distributed in a continuous smear from the position of the form I band to the late Cairns structure band. Replication of form I SV40 DNA begins with unwinding of the parental DNA strands to form a small replication bubble at the origin of replication. The replication bubble then grows, progressively increasing the size and decreasing the compactness of the replication intermediate. When the intermediate is about 95% replicated, it is a late Cairns structure which is about twice the size of the original chromosome and completely relaxed. Single strand DNA breaks relax intermediate Cairns structures. These "nicked Cairns structures" have greatly reduced electrophoretic mobility since they are not as compact as the superhelical Cairns intermediates. Nicked Cairns replication intermediates are distributed as a continuous smear from the position of the form II band to the position of the late Cairns structure. This is logical. Nicks convert form I to form II and so will convert the earliest Cairns structure from a form I molecule with a very small replication bubble, thus migrating at a position just behind form I, to a form II molecule with a small replication bubble, migrating at a position just behind form II. The topological structure and electrophoretic mobility of the late Cairns structure, however, is not affected by nicking. This means that the late Cairns structure is normally relaxed. The linkage deficit of early replication intermediates is removed by the end of DNA replication.

COLLISION OF DNA REPLICATION FORKS WITH DRUG-STABILIZED TOPOISOMERASE I-DNA STRAND PASSING COMPLEXES

Topoisomerase I changes the topology of DNA by introducing transient single strand DNA breaks through which the remaining strand of the DNA helix is passed. The enzyme is covalently attached to the DNA on the 3' side of the DNA strand break during the strand passing reaction (Fig. 3.1). Camptothecin is a very cytotoxic natural product from the Chinese plant *Camptotheca acuminata.* Camptothecin and its analogs are topoisomerase I poisons which stabilize cleavable complexes, topoisomerase I reaction intermediates in which the enzyme is covalently attached to the DNA at the site of a DNA strand break.[8] Addition of a protein denaturant will convert this "cleavable complex" into a permanent, protein-associated DNA strand break. Since strong protein denaturants are not present in cells, it was originally not clear why the reversible stabilization of this reaction intermediate should be so cytotoxic. When the drug diffuses away from the cleavable complex, the topoisomerase completes its strand passing reaction without leaving any DNA damage.

CAMPTOTHECIN EXPOSURE CAUSES DOUBLE STRAND DNA BREAKS AT SV40 DNA REPLICATION FORKS

When camptothecin is added to SV40-infected cells, normal replication intermediates are instantly replaced by aberrant forms.[9] In one-dimensional agarose gel electrophoresis patterns these aberrant forms include two short smears of replication intermediates (LC' and LC'') located in the region between the late Cairns structure and the form II band. Camptothecin exposure also causes an intensification of the form III DNA band. Long fluorographic exposures revealed a smear (III') extending from the form III band. Two dimensional neutral-alkaline gel electrophoresis shows these smears as arcs of nascent strands[9-11] with LC' being asymptotic to the first dimension gel position of form II and LC'' being asymptotic to the first dimension gel position of form III (Fig. 3.3). This indicates that forms II and III represent the "zero percent replicated" forms of these intermediates (see chapter 2). Two-dimensional neutral-alkaline and neutral-chloroquine gel electrophoresis patterns of camptothecin-induced aberrant SV40 DNA replication intermediates are diagrammed in Figure 3.4. These aberrant intermediates, with one exception discussed below, can be produced by partial S1 nuclease digestion of normal SV40 DNA replication intermediates.[12] S1 nuclease is a single strand specific nuclease which rapidly digests the single strand regions of replication forks. The partially digested forms produced will have double strand DNA breaks at one or more replication forks.

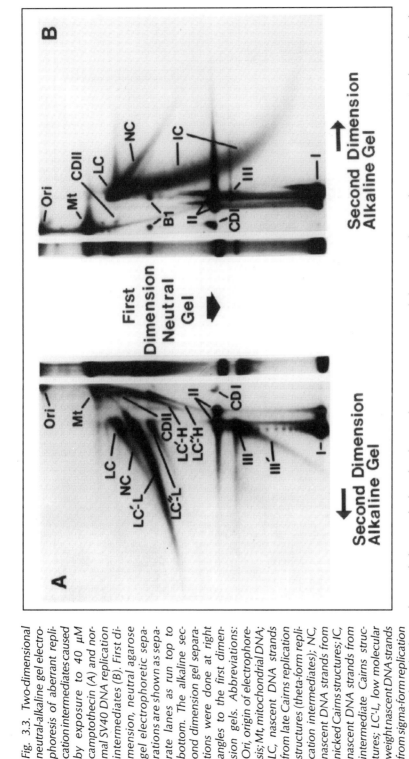

Fig. 3.3. Two-dimensional neutral-alkaline gel electrophoresis of aberrant replication intermediates caused by exposure to 40 µM camptothecin (A) and normal SV40 DNA replication intermediates (B). First dimension, neutral agarose gel electrophoretic separations are shown as separate lanes as run from top to bottom. The alkaline second dimension gel separations were done at right angles to the first dimension gels. Abbreviations: Ori, origin of electrophoresis; Mt, mitochondrial DNA; LC, nascent DNA strands from late Cairns replication structures (theta-form replication intermediates); NC, nascent DNA strands from nicked Cairns structures; IC, nascent DNA strands from intermediate Cairns structures; LC'L, low molecular weight nascent DNA strands from sigma-form replication structures with one broken replication fork; LC'H, high molecular weight nascent DNA strands from sigma-form replication structures; LC"L, low molecular weight nascent DNA strands from replication structures linearized by two replication fork breaks; LC"H, high molecular weight nascent DNA strands from replication structures; II, newly synthesized DNA strands from form II (nicked circle) SV40 genomes; III, newly synthesized DNA strands from form III (double strand linear) SV40 genomes; III', nascent strands from replication bubbles detached by two replication fork breaks; CDII, form I circular (head-to-tail dimer); CDI, form II (nicked) circular dimer; B1, B-family catenated dimer; I, form I (superhelical) SV40 DNA. Catenated dimers are discussed in chapter 4 and circular dimers are discussed in chapter 8. In B, CDI is not resolved from C-family catenated dimers. The horizontal streaks extending from forms II, III and LC in the alkaline second dimension are indications of single strand breaks in the nascent DNA strands. The "knob" on the form I DNA spot is form II DNA produced by radiolytic nicking of the heavily labeled form I DNA during preparation for the alkaline second dimension electrophoresis.

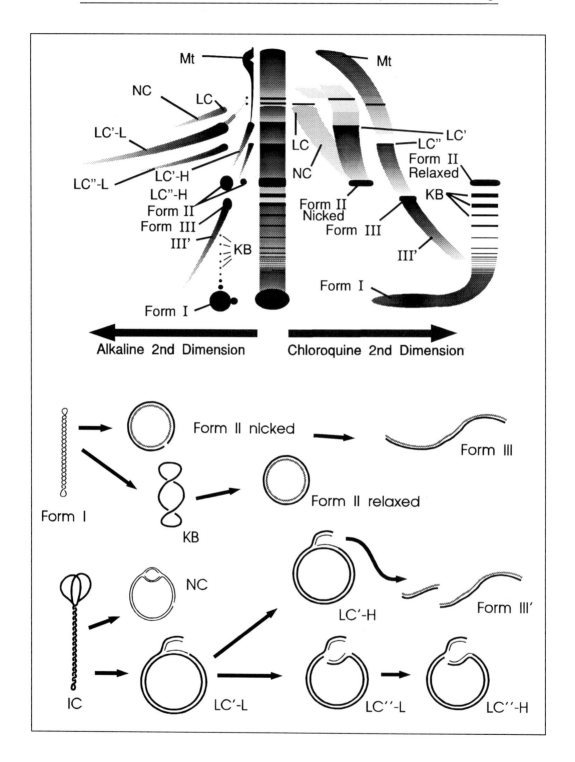

CAMPTOTHECIN-INDUCED DNA REPLICATION FORK BREAKAGE OCCURS BY COLLISIONS WITH DRUG-STABILIZED TOPOISOMERASE I-DNA CLEAVABLE COMPLEXES ON EITHER LEADING OR LAGGING STRAND SIDES

The LC' intermediates are "sigma" forms which resemble rolling circles. They are not true rolling circles since they do not have multimeric tails. These LC' intermediates are produced by breakage of a parental DNA strand at one replication fork. The mechanism of fork breakage is collision of the replication fork with the drug-stabilized topoisomerase I-DNA cleavage complex (Fig. 3.5). The LC' intermediates are linear forms resulting from two replication fork breaks, and the III' forms are detached replication bubbles resulting from two replication fork breaks on the same parental DNA strand but on opposite sides of the replication bubble. The increase in intensity of the form III band upon exposure to camptothecin is due to detachment of replication bubbles from

Fig. 3.4. (on opposite page) Diagram of two-dimensional neutral-alkaline and neutral-chloroquine agarose gel electrophoresis patterns of camptothecin-induced aberrant SV40 DNA replication intermediates. The first dimension neutral electrophoresis is shown in the top middle as run from top to bottom. The alkaline second dimension is shown as run to the left and the chloroquine second dimension is to the right of the first dimension lane. KB, Keller bands (covalently closed form I DNA with low levels of supercoiling). Other abbreviations are the same as in Figure 3.3. Keller bands are not part of the camptothecin pattern of aberrant replication intermediates but are included here since they can be seen in Figure 3.3. Pronounced Keller bands are often due to inhibition of protein synthesis which prevents the formation of nucleosomes on newly replicated daughter chromosomes. Keller bands can be made by partial relaxation of form I DNA with topoisomerase I. In the lower half of the figure, a single strand break converts form I DNA to nicked form II, and a double strand break converts it to form III. Partial relaxation of form I gives Keller band intermediates, and complete relaxation gives relaxed form II (covalently closed). In the same way, a nick in a parental DNA strand converts superhelical intermediate Cairns structures (IC) to nicked Cairns structures. A single, broken replication fork converts intermediate Cairns structures to LC'-L in which the nascent strands range in size from short oligonucleotides to full SV40 genome length. These are converted to LC'-H by the covalent attachment of nascent strands to parental strands at the site of the fork break. The unlabeled parental strand is full genome length, so covalent attachment of labeled nascent strands results in a family of high molecular weight labeled strands ranging in size from one to two SV40 genome lengths. A secondary replication fork break in LC'-L or LC'-H can detach a replication bubble to generate form III', a family of subgenomic double strand linear DNAs. A second replication fork break in LC'-L can also generate LC''-L linear forms with labeled nascent strands ranging in size from small oligonucleotides to full genome length single strand DNA. Ligation of one of the nascent strands to a parental strand gives LC''-H with high molecular weight nascent strands ranging from one to two SV40 genome lengths.

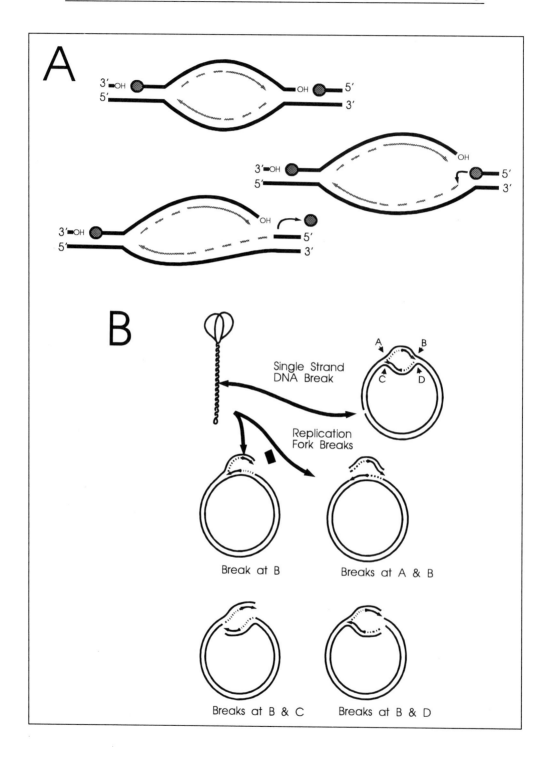

the heavily labeled late Cairns structures.[12] Since these structures are approximately 95% replicated, the detached replication bubbles are essentially full length linear SV40 DNA and are thus not well resolved from true form III molecules. Detachment of replication bubbles means that replication fork breaks have occurred on both leading and lagging strand sides of the replication forks (see Fig. 3.5, A).

Exposure to camptothecin causes immediate breakage of at least one DNA replication fork on every replication intermediate.[9] If topoisomerase I were acting randomly on the unreplicated region, nicked Cairns structures would be the expected result of camptothecin exposure. Yet, the only intact replication intermediates seen after camptothecin-treatment are a trace of late Cairns structures. The rapid and extensive breakage of SV40 DNA replication forks by camptothecin treatment suggests that topoisomerase I is acting at or just ahead of the replication forks. Such localization implies that topoisomerase I may be part of the multiprotein replication complex (MRC). Recombinant SV40 large T antigen has been reported to have a topoisomerase I activity,[13,14] and the same has been found for polyomavirus large T antigen.[15] Thus, topoisomerase I either binds very tightly to large T antigen or the large T antigen itself has a topoisomerase I activity. Since large T antigen is the helicase for unwinding of the replication origin and may be the helicase for replication of the entire viral genome, this association can potentially account for the rapid, extensive breakage of replication forks by camptothecin. Topisomerase I is a component of the mammalian DNA replication complex as well (chapter 7).

Fig. 3.5. (on opposite page) Mechanism of camptothecin-induced SV40 DNA replication fork breakage. (A.) Replication forks approach camptothecin-stabilized topoisomerase I-DNA cleavable complexes on both the leading and lagging strand sides. A double strand break occurs when the leading strand side of the right fork meets a cleavable complex. The subsequent ligation of nascent strands to parental strands may be mediated by the topoisomerase I as shown. Extensive detachment of replication bubbles in SV40 intermediates from camptothecin-treated cells indicates that a double strand break also occurs when the left fork meets a camptothecin-stabilized cleavable complex. This is a break on the lagging strand side. (B.) Combinations of replication fork breaks to produce aberrant SV40 intermediates. Forms with breaks at B and D have not been detected in two-dimensional gel patterns. If they occur, they are either rare or hidden in the LC'-L arc.

NEWLY SYNTHESIZED NASCENT DNA STRANDS BECOME
COVALENTLY ATTACHED TO PARENTAL DNA STRANDS
IN A SIGNIFICANT FRACTION OF THE REPLICATION
INTERMEDIATES WITH BROKEN REPLICATION FORKS

As mentioned above, partial S1 nuclease digestion of the single strand DNA gaps at replication forks produces a pattern of aberrant SV40 intermediates similar to those caused by camptothecin exposure to infected cells. There is one difference between the pattern of aberrant intermediates produced by camptothecin treatment and that produced by S1 nuclease digestion of normal SV40 intermediates. Second dimension alkaline gel electrophoresis of viral DNA from camptothecin-treated cells separates the LC' and LC'' smears into high and low molecular weight arcs (Figs. 3.3 and 3.4). Only the lower molecular weight arcs (LC'-L and LC''-L) are present in the S1 nuclease digestion products.[12] The LC'-L and LC''-L arcs seen on two dimensional neutral-alkaline gel patterns are due to nascent strands detached under the alkaline conditions of the second dimension. In the alkaline second dimension these arcs extend from a point ahead of the dye front to the level of full length linear DNA (marked by the form III spot). The nascent strands from the earliest replication intermediates (normal or aberrant) are derived from very small replication bubbles and are thus very short oligonucleotides. These short nascent strands are expected to migrate rapidly through the gel. Nascent strands from nearly completed late replication intermediates are approximately full SV40 genome length single strand DNAs. Thus nascent strands from sigma forms and linear forms caused by replication fork breaks are expected to form arcs extending from ahead of the dye front to the level of full length linear DNA in the alkaline second dimension.

The high molecular weight LC' and LC'' arcs (LC'-H and LC''-H), seen only in the DNA from camptothecin-treated cells, extend from the level of full length linear SV40 DNA to the level of double length genomes. Since these are not produced by S1 digestion, they are not simple products of replication fork breakage. These upper arcs are seen only under the denaturing conditions of the alkaline second dimension gel—conditions which normally separate labeled nascent strands from unlabeled parental DNA

strands. The subsets of intermediates making up the LC'-H and
LC''-H arcs are indistinguishable from those making up the LC'-L
and LC''-L arcs under the nondenaturing conditions of the first
dimension electrophoresis. This means that they are sigma and linear forms, respectively. The mechanism for formation of these upper or high molecular weight LC'-H and LC''-H arcs is covalent
attachment of a nascent strand to a parental strand at the site of a
DNA fork break (Fig. 3.5, A). The parental DNA strand is full
genome length SV40 DNA. If nascent strands from early replication bubbles become attached to one of these parental DNA
strands, the resulting strand would be only slightly longer than
full length linear SV40 DNA. At the other extreme, if the nascent
strand from an almost completely replicated late Cairns structure
becomes covalently attached to a parental DNA strand, the resulting strand is approximately two SV40 genome lengths. This is the
simplest explanation for the high molecular weight LC'-H and
LC''-H arcs seen in samples from camptothecin-treated cells. This
mechanism also explains why the upper arcs are not seen in the
S1 nuclease digestion products of normal intermediates: the S1
nuclease can cause breaks at replication forks, but cannot ligate
DNA strands. In camptothecin-treated cells, the ligation event may
be carried out by the covalently attached topoisomerase I molecule as indicated in Figure 3.5, A. Attachment of a nascent strand
to a parental strand is a recombinational event and can be seen as
a partially completed sister chromatid exchange.[9]

   There is evidence of other camptothecin-induced recombinational events in SV40 DNA. In two-dimensional neutral-alkaline
gel patterns, a faint extension can be seen running from the top
of the lower LC' arc to a small spot located behind the late Cairns
structure in the first dimension and at about the level of double
length linear SV40 DNA in the second dimension. This streak is
thick near the upper end of the LC' arc and abruptly thins
(Figs. 3.3 and 3.4). The nature of the intermediates giving rise to
these elements of the gel pattern are not known. They are not
seen in the S1 nuclease digestion products of normal intermediates.[12] The spot at the upper end of the extension is in the general
area of the late Cairns structure, the A-1 catenated dimer, and the
circular head-to-tail dimer. All of these are approximately double

sized circular SV40 DNA forms. These aberrant forms are associated with the LC' arc in two-dimensional neutral-chloroquine gel electrophoresis patterns of camptothecin-induced aberrant SV40 replication intermediates (Fig. 3.6). This suggests that they may be related to or derived from sigma forms with broken replication forks.

The breakage of SV40 DNA replication forks by camptothecin has been confirmed by similar studies done with electron microscopy rather than two-dimensional gel electrophoresis.[16] Replication

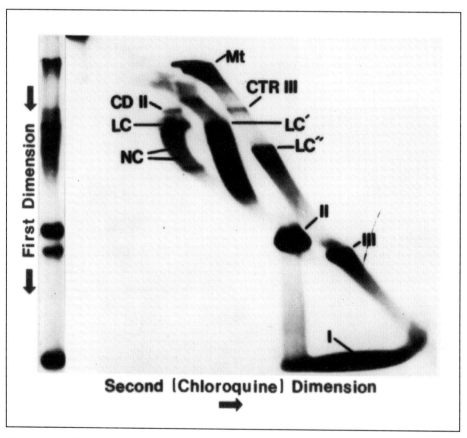

Fig. 3.6. *Two-dimensional neutral-chloroquine gel electrophoresis of aberrant SV40 intermediates from camptothecin-treated infected cells. The abbreviations and structures for the aberrant forms are given in Figure 3.4. The forms extending upward from the arc of LC' forms are not seen in similar intermediates produced by S1 nuclease digestion of normal SV40 DNA replication intermediates. This suggests that they are recombinational in nature and not simple products of replication fork breaks. CTRIII, circular trimer form III. Other abbreviations are the same as in Figures 3.3 and 3.4. (P. Permana, unpublished data).*

fork breakage by collision with camptothecin-stabilized topo-isomerase I-DNA cleavable complexes has also been confirmed using an in vitro SV40 DNA replication system.[17] In the in vitro repli-cation system replication fork breaks occurred only on the leading strand sides of replication forks. The detachment of SV40 DNA replication bubbles by in vivo camptothecin treatment shows that fork breaks do occur to a significant extent on both leading and lagging strand sides of replication forks in intact cells.[12] However, the kinetics of replication fork breakage shows that single fork breaks occur much more rapidly than the double replication fork breaks that detach replication bubbles.[18] This suggests that repli-cation fork breaks may occur more readily in one orientation, prob-ably on the leading strand side. Preferential breakage on leading strand sides of forks can be rationalized in terms of the model shown in Figure 3.5. When meeting drug-stabilized topoisomerase I cleavable complexes on the leading strand side, the replication fork will encounter the single strand DNA break first. On the lagging strand side it must encounter the covalently attached en-zyme first, and this might slow the fork breakage. However, the in vivo studies with SV40 clearly show extensive detachment of replication bubbles even at early times after drug exposure. This means that lagging strand replication fork breaks occur to a sig-nificant extent in vivo and are likely to contribute to the cytotox-icity of camptothecin in mammalian cells. The slower kinetics of replication bubble detachment compared to the formation of sigma replication forms may just reflect the kinetics of two events versus the kinetics of one event.

DNA POLYMERASE INHIBITION

Inhibition of DNA polymerase also causes dramatic changes in the structure and electrophoretic mobility of SV40 DNA replica-tion intermediates. Aphidicolin inhibits both DNA polymerases delta and alpha, which are thought to be the leading and lagging strand polymerases, respectively, of the mammalian replication fork.[19-21] When aphidicolin is added to SV40-infected cells, the late and intermediate Cairns replication intermediates undergo pro-nounced changes in structure which increase their electrophoretic mobility.[22,23] The electrophoretic mobility of these Cairns structures increases progressively with continuing exposure to aphidicolin[23] until the entire range of Cairns replication intermediates is compressed into a broad band which migrates just behind the form I band on one dimensional agarose gels. These compact, torsionally stressed replication intermediates are termed 40S intermediates since they sediment collectively at that rate in sucrose gradients.[22]

The 40S intermediates appear as a compressed arc on two-dimensional neutral-alkaline gel electrophoresis.[23] On two dimensional neutral-chloroquine gels, the 40S intermediates appear as a short diagonal extending from the right end of the form I spot to a position directly above it (Fig. 3.7). The 40S intermediates are unstable and spontaneously break down in vivo with the formation of DNA strand breaks and protein-DNA crosslinks (Fig. 3.8).[23] This nicking converts the 40S intermediates to nicked Cairns structures which are crosslinked to protein (Fig. 3.9). A fraction of the form II and III DNA is crosslinked to protein as is some higher molecular weight DNA found in the region of the mitochondrial DNA band after 40S breakdown. The 40S intermediates themselves are not crosslinked to protein.

Exposure to aphidicolin permanently inactivates SV40 replication intermediates.[24,25] Consistent with this, there is no repair of the DNA strand breaks or protein-DNA crosslinks in the nicked Cairns structures resulting from 40S breakdown.[23] Although they do not replicate again, the damaged SV40 replication intermediates undergo progressive changes with time after aphidicolin exposure. Following the relatively rapid 40S breakdown to nicked Cairns structures, the replication intermediates undergo replication fork breakage to produce LC' forms which resolve into LC'-L and LC'-H arcs in neutral-chloroquine two-dimensional gel separations. Eventually an LC''-H arc is formed without an LC''-L arc, and the bulk of the labeled viral DNA becomes progressively higher in molecular weight. These changes occur either during a chase with unlabeled thymidine or in the continued presence of 60 μM aphidicolin. This rules out involvement of DNA synthesis in the structural changes that must be recombinational in nature. The high molecular weight forms remained crosslinked to protein. The recombinational events following 40S breakdown appear to take a different pathway from those following camptothecin exposure.

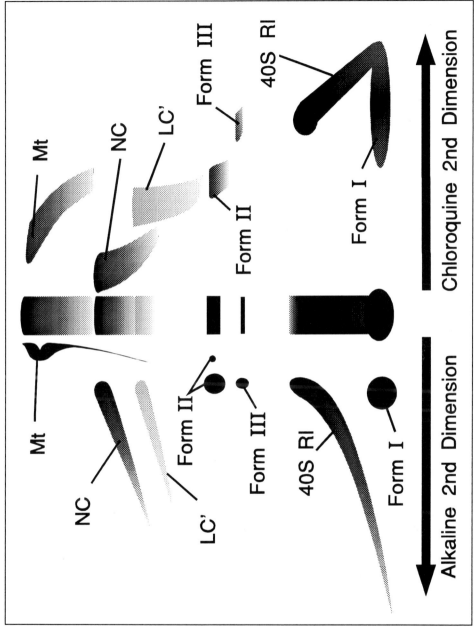

Fig. 3.7. Diagram of two-dimensional neutral-alkaline and neutral-chloroquine electrophoresis patterns resulting from exposure of infected cells to aphidicolin. 40S RI, compact, torsionally stressed replication intermediates. As shown in the alkaline second dimension, the full range of nascent strands is present. Other abbreviations are the same as in Figures 3.3 and 3.4.

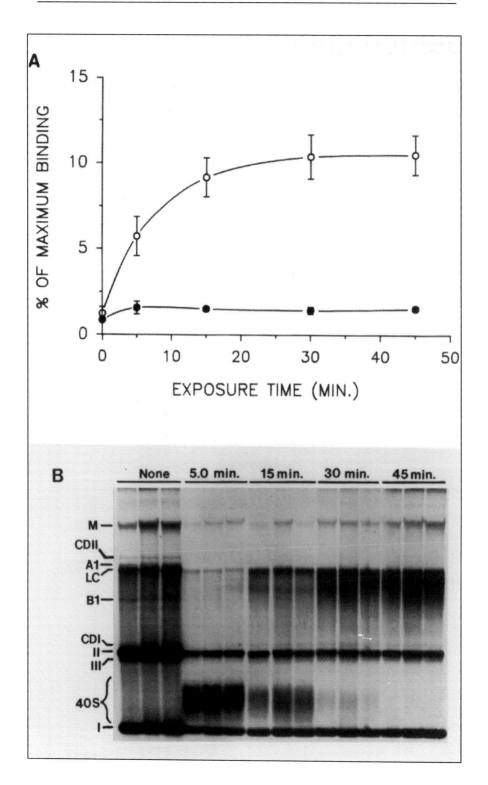

The 40S intermediates begin to break down as they are being formed. This is indicated by low-level protein-DNA crosslinking immediately after aphidicolin exposure. However, formation of 40S intermediates is more rapid than their breakdown so that a substantial temporary accumulation of 40S intermediates occurs. Protein-DNA crosslinks reach a maximum as nicking of the 40S intermediates is completed in the somewhat slower breakdown phase. A slower secondary breakdown occurs over the next 24 hours as the inactivated Cairns structures with protein-associated DNA strand breaks undergo additional structural changes which increase their size in the absence of DNA replication. Alkaline two-dimensional gel analysis of this very slow second phase breakdown suggests recombinational changes, including ligations of nascent strands to parental strands.[23] Since topoisomerases cause protein-associated DNA strand breaks during their reaction cycles, we speculate that the 40S intermediate may be a suicide substrate for a cellular topoisomerase.

STRUCTURE OF 40S INTERMEDIATES

The late replication forms undergo the most pronounced structural changes during formation of 40S intermediates. The electrophoretic mobility of the late Cairns structure in first dimension, neutral agarose gel electrophoresis is greatly increased while the

Fig. 3.8. (on opposite page) The spontaneous nicking of newly formed 40S intermediates is accompanied by protein crosslinking to the SV40 DNA. SV40-infected cells were labeled with tritiated thymidine at the peak of viral DNA replication, 36 hr post-infection. Aphidicolin (60 μM) was added to the labeling medium 15 min after the start of labeling. Hirt extractions were done on the cells at the drug exposure times indicated. Aliquots of each Hirt supernatant were removed for protein-DNA crosslink assays, either with or without prior proteinase K digestion. The remainder of each sample was deproteinized and prepared for one-dimensional, neutral agarose gel electrophoresis. (A.) Protein-DNA crosslinks as measured by the GF/C filter assay (chapter 2). Samples predigested with proteinase K, ○; samples assayed directly for protein-DNA crosslinks, ●. The percentage of maximum binding is the percentage of pulse-labeled viral intermediates crosslinked to protein. Error bars are standard deviations. (B.) One dimensional, agarose gel electrophoresis of SV40 DNA replication intermediates from aphidicolin-treated cells. Experiments were done in triplicate for gel electrophoresis. A1, A-family catenated dimer with catenation linking number of 1. Other abbreviations are the same as in Figures 3.3 and 3.4. The darkening of the contaminating mitochondrial DNA band at 45 min is due largely to the additive effect of other labeled intermediates accumulating in the region between the late Cairns structure (LC) and the loading slot. Reprinted from Nucleic Acids Res 1991; 19:5065 by permission of Oxford University Press.

Fig. 3.9. GF/C filter elution of SV40 forms crosslinked to protein during the formation and breakdown of aphidicolin-induced 40S intermediates. Lanes 1-4; Aliquots taken from Hirt extract supernatants, deproteinized and prepared for electrophoresis. Aliquots from pulse-labeled untreated cells (lane 1), from cells treated with 60 µM aphidicolin for 3 and 45 min (lanes 2 and 3), and from cells treated with aphidicolin for 45 min, then chased with unlabeled thymidine for 24 hr (lane 4). Lanes 5-6; Aliquots from the Hirt supernatants used for lanes 1-5 were adjusted to 0.4 M guanidinium chloride and passed through pre-wetted GF/C glass fiber filters. Only DNA crosslinked to protein is bound to the glass fiber filter in 0.4 M guanidinium chloride. These forms were eluted from the filters in a buffer composed of 10 mM Tris HCl, pH 7.5, 1.0 mM NaEDTA, 100 mM NaCl, 0.1% SDS. The eluted samples were deproteinzed by digestion with proteinase K before electrophoresis. Normal SV40 DNA replication intermediates (lanes 1 and 5) and 40S intermediates (lanes 2 and 6) are not bound to

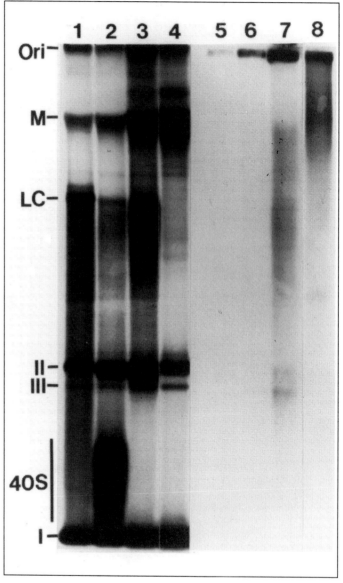

the filter and, therefore, have no protein-DNA crosslinks. After spontaneous in vivo breakdown by nicking (lanes 3 and 7), the replication intermediates are crosslinked to protein. Some form II and III DNA is also crosslinked to protein as is some of the higher molecular weight DNA migrating more slowly than the late Cairns structure (LC). At longer times after aphidicolin exposure, only high molecular weight DNA is crosslinked to protein (lanes 4 and 8). If aliquots are digested with proteinase K before GF/C filtration, nothing is bound or eluted (not shown). Abbreviations same as in Figures 3.3, 3.4 and 3.7. Reprinted from Nucleic Acids Res 1991; 19:5065 by permission of Oxford University Press.

electrophoretic mobility of early replication intermediates is almost unaffected. This causes the entire range of replication intermediates to migrate in a thick band just behind the form I band in such one-dimensional gels. Since single strand DNA breaks convert 40S forms to nicked Cairns structures, the basis of the structural change must be superhelicity. The model for 40S formation, involving re-annealing of replication forks with extended single strand regions, suggests that this is very high negative superhelicity. The more pronounced compaction of late replication structures can be understood if it is assumed that differences in parental DNA strand linkage can be distributed between superhelicity in the unreplicated region and intertwining of double strands in the replicated region (Fig. 3.10). In late replication structures, most of the linkage deficit would have to be distributed into the replicated region. The electron microscopy studies of Dröge and coworkers demonstrated intertwining of the replicated region in 40S intermediates.[22]

At the other extreme, the linkage deficit would have to be almost entirely distributed into the unreplicated region in early replication intermediates with very small replication bubbles. Since this region is normally superhelical, the additional superhelicity associated with 40S intermediates might not increase compaction significantly. This would explain why the electrophoretic mobility of early 40S intermediates is not significantly changed in the first dimension, neutral agarose gel electrophoresis conditions. However, second dimension, chloroquine gel electrophoresis shows that even the early intermediates have greatly altered superhelicity. The earliest normal Cairns structures migrate more slowly than the bulk of form I, and the earliest 40S intermediates migrate more rapidly than bulk form I DNA in the chloroquine second dimension. This behavior alone does not distinguish between increased or decreased negative superhelicity in the 40S intermediates. If the 40S intermediates were less superhelical than normal intermediate Cairns structures, chloroquine could cause significant positive supercoiling and increase their electrophoretic mobility as it does with relaxed form II DNA. However, decreased negative superhelicity in Cairns structures makes them less compact and decreases their electrophoretic mobility in neutral first dimension agarose gel electrophoresis—the opposite of what is seen. The evidence thus favors very high level negative superhelicity in the 40S intermediates. It is likely that the negative superhelicity is so high that the 40S intermediates cannot be relaxed by the concentration of chloroquine used in the standard second dimension chloroquine gel electrophoresis.

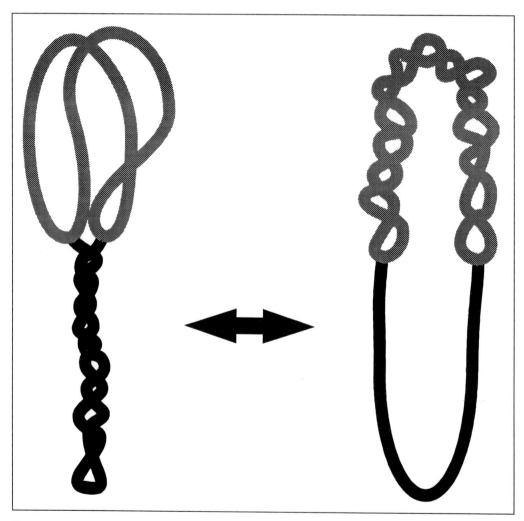

Fig. 3.10. Interconversion of parental DNA strand linkage between superhelicity in the unreplicated region and intertwining in the replicated region of an intermediate Cairns structure. Two extremes are shown. The replicated daughter strands are shown in gray and the unreplicated region in black.

SV40 REPLICATION FORK INSTABILITY
AND MAMMALIAN REPLICONS

Do mammalian replication forks undergo similar damage when cells in S-phase are exposed to agents like camptothecin and aphidicolin? There is substantial evidence supporting the idea that camptothecin damages mammalian replication forks much as it does SV40 replication forks. Aphidicolin exposure reduces the cytotoxicity of camptothecin significantly.[26,27] It is thought that it does this by arresting fork movement and preventing collisions with the camptothecin-stabilized topoisomerase I-DNA cleavable complexes. There is also evidence of S-phase specific DNA double strand breaks caused by camptothecin, presumably at replication forks.[28,29]

There is no evidence that aphidicolin causes replication fork collapse or replicon inactivation in mammalian chromosomes. There are no reports of protein-DNA crosslinks following aphidicolin treatment of uninfected mammalian cells. Our search for such crosslinks has been completely negative. The model for 40S formation involves arrest of DNA polymerase while DNA helicases and topoisomerases continue to unwind the parental DNA strands to create extended single stranded regions. The fact that protein-DNA crosslinks and bulky alkylating agents can also cause 40S intermediates (chapter 5) is consistent with this model if it is assumed that these bulky DNA adducts are able to block DNA polymerase movement without significant inhibition of DNA helicase or topoisomerases. Arrest of DNA polymerase movement may be indirect, by blocking accessory proteins or "sliding clamps" associated with the polymerases. The SV40 large T antigen is known to be a DNA helicase.[30-34] It unwinds the parental DNA strands to open a replication bubble at the SV40 origin of replication and may act as a helicase throughout SV40 DNA replication. Cyclobutane pyrimidine dimers have been reported to efficiently block SV40 DNA synthesis in vitro while having negligible effect on large T antigen helicase activity.[35] Cellular DNA helicases may be more tightly associated with other enzymes of the DNA replication complex. If so, the question arises: "could genetic instability in mammalian cells be caused by mutant DNA helicases with loose connections to other proteins of the replication complex?" A recent report suggests a connection between genetic instability and helicases. The mutated *BLM* gene responsible for Bloom's syndrome, an inherited human disease of genetic instability, has been reported to have significant homology to known DNA helicases.[36] Several lines of evidence suggest that the normal *BLM* gene may play some role in DNA replication.

If the 40S pathway of replication fork collapse is uniquely associated with the viral large T antigen, there is a possibility that DNA replication in other papovaviruses may be susceptible to similar disruption. Since replication fork collapse by the 40S pathway is associated with recombinational events, this type of genetic instability may be involved in integration into cellular chromosomes and rearrangements of the viral chromosomes. Oncogenic transformation by papovaviruses typically involves such rearrangements and integration into cellular chromosomes. Drugs and agents causing 40S pathway replication arrest in papovaviruses may thus be oncogenic only in papovavirus-infected cells.

REFERENCES

1. White JH, Gallo R, Bauer WR. Effect of nucleosome distortion on the linking deficiency in relaxed minichromosomes. J Mol Biol 1989; 207:193-199.
2. Patterton H-G, Von Holt C. Negative supercoiling and nucleosome cores. I. The effect of negative supercoiling on the efficiency of nucleosome core formation in vitro. J Mol Biol 1993; 229:623-636.
3. Germond JE, Hirt B, Oudet P et al. Folding of the DNA double helix in chromatin-like structures from simian virus 40. Proc Natl Acad Sci USA 1975; 72:1843-1847.
4. Been MD, Champoux JJ. Topoisomerases and the swivel problem. In: Alberts B, Fox CF, eds. Mechanistic studies of DNA replication and genetic recombination. New York: Academic Press, Inc. 1980:809-815.
5. Sebring ED, Garon CF, Salzman NP. Superhelix density of replicating simian virus 40 DNA molecules. J Mol Biol 1974; 90:371-379.
6. Salzman NP, Lebowitz J, Chen M et al. Properties of replicating SV40 DNA molecules and mapping unpaired regions in SV40 DNA I. Cold Spring Harbor Symp Quant Biol 1975; 39:209-218.
7. Jaenisch R, Levine A. DNA replication in SV40-infected cells. V. Circular and catenated oligomers of SV40 DNA. Virology 1971; 44:480-493.

8. Hsiang Y-H, Hertzberg R, Hecht S et al. Camptothecin induces protein-linked DNA breaks via mammalian DNA topoisomerase I. J Biol Chem 1985; 260:14873-14878.

9. Snapka RM. Topoisomerase inhibitors can selectively interfere with different stages of simian virus 40 DNA replication. Mol Cell Biol 1986; 6:4221-4227.

10. Snapka RM, Permana PA. SV40 DNA replication intermediates: analysis of drugs which target mammalian DNA replication. BioEssays 1993; 15:121-127.

11. Snapka RM, Permana PA, Marquit G et al. Two-dimensional agarose gel analysis of simian virus 40 DNA replication intermediates. Methods: A Companion to Methods in Enzymology 1991; 3:73-82.

12. Shin C-G, Snapka RM. Exposure to camptothecin breaks leading and lagging strand simian virus 40 DNA replication forks. Biochem Biophys Res Commun 1990; 168:135-140.

13. Marton A, Jean D, Delbecchi L et al. Topoisomerase activity associated with SV40 large tumor antigen. Nucleic Acids Res 1993; 21:1689-1695.

14. Mann K. Topoisomerase activity is associated with purified SV40 T antigen. Nucleic Acids Res 1993; 21:1697-1704.

15. Marton A, Marko B, Delbecchi L et al. Topoisomerase activity associated with polyoma virus large tumor antigen. Biochim Biophys Acta Gene Struct Expression 1995; 1262:59-63.

16. Avemann K, Knippers R, Koller T et al. Camptothecin, a specific inhibitor of type I DNA topoisomerase, induces DNA breakage at replication forks. Mol Cell Biol 1988; 8:3026-3034.

17. Tsao Y-P, Russo A, Nyamuswa G et al. Interaction between replication forks and topoisomerase I-DNA cleavable complexes: Studies in a cell-free SV40 DNA replication system. Cancer Res 1993; 53:5908-5914.

18. Snapka RM, Powelson MA, Strayer JM. Swiveling and decatenation of replicating simian virus 40 genomes in vivo. Mol Cell Biol 1988; 8:515-521.

19. Spadari S, Sala F, Pedrali-Noy G. Aphidicolin and eukaryotic DNA synthesis. Adv Exp Med Biol 1984; 179:169-181.

20. Haraguchi T, Uguro M, Nagano H et al. Specific inhibitors of eukaryotic DNA synthesis and DNA polymerase alpha. Nucleic Acids Res 1983; 11:1197-1209.

21. Goulian M, Heard CJ. An inhibitor of DNA polymerases α and δ in calf thymus DNA. Nucleic Acids Res 1990; 18:4791-4796.

22. Dröge P, Sogo JM, Stahl H. Inhibition of DNA synthesis by aphidicolin induces supercoiling in simian virus 40 replicative intermediates. EMBO J 1985; 4:3241-3246.

23. Snapka RM, Shin C-G, Permana PA et al. Aphidicolin-induced topological and recombinational events in simian virus 40. Nucleic Acids Res 1991; 19:5065-5072.

24. Dinter-Gottlieb G, Kaufmann G. Aphidicolin arrest irreversibly impairs replicating simian virus 40 chromosomes. J Biol Chem 1983; 258:3809-3812.

25. Nethanel T, Reisfeld S, Dinter-Gottlieb G et al. An Okazaki piece of simian virus 40 may be synthesized by ligation of shorter precursor chains. J Virol 1988; 62:2867-2873.

26. Holm C, Covey JM, Kerrigan D et al. Differential requirement of DNA replication for the cytotoxicity of DNA topoisomerase I and II inhibitors in Chinese hamster DC3F cells. Cancer Res 1989; 49:6365-6368.

27. Hsiang Y-H, Lihou MG, Liu LF. Arrest of replication forks by drug-stabilized topoisomerase I-DNA cleavable complexes as a mechanism of cell killing by camptothecin. Cancer Res 1989; 49:5077-5082.

28. Squires S, Ryan AJ, Strutt HL et al. Deoxyguanosine enhances the cytotoxicity of the topoisomerase I inhibitor camptothecin by reducing the repair of double-strand breaks induced in replicating DNA. J Cell Science 1991; 100:883-893.

29. Ryan AJ, Squires S, Strutt HL et al. Camptothecin cytotoxicity in mammalian cells is associated with the induction of persistent double strand breaks in replicating DNA. Nucleic Acids Res 1991; 19:3295-3300.

30. Parsons R, Anderson ME, Tegtmeyer P. Three domains in the simian virus 40 core origin orchestrate the binding, melting, and DNA helicase activities of T antigen. J Virol 1990; 64:509-518.

31. Borowiec JA, Dean FB, Bullock PA et al. Binding and unwinding—how T antigen engages the SV40 origin of DNA replication. Cell 1990; 60:181-184.

32. Wun-Kim K, Simmons DT. Mapping of helicase and helicase substrate-binding domains on simian virus 40 large T antigen. J Virol 1990; 64:2014-2020.

33. Stahl H, Dröge P, Knippers R. DNA helicase activity of SV40 large tumor antigen. EMBO J 1986; 5:1939-1944.

34. Yang L, Jessee CB, Lau K et al. Template supercoiling during ATP-dependent DNA helix tracking: Studies with simian virus 40 large tumor antigen. Proc Natl Acad Sci USA 1989; 86:6121-6125.

35. Gough G, Wood RD. Inhibition of in vitro SV40 DNA replication by ultraviolet light. Mutat Res 1989; 227:193-197.

36. Ellis NA, Groden J, Ye T-Z et al. The Bloom's syndrome gene product is homologous to RecQ helicases. Cell 1995; 83:655-666.

CHAPTER 4

TOPOISOMERASE II AND TERMINATION OF DNA REPLICATION

Robert M. Snapka and Edith F. Yamasaki

THE TERMINATION PROBLEM

The linkage of DNA strands in a circular double stranded DNA like the SV40 chromosome presents two closely related problems in DNA replication: the swivel problem and the linkage problem. The swivel problem was discussed in chapter 3 and refers to the need to continually reduce parental DNA strand linkage so that positive superhelical stress in the unreplicated region does not prevent replication fork movement. This chapter will focus on the termination problem—reducing parental DNA strand linkage to zero so that daughter chromosomes can separate. The parental DNA strands are topologically linked once for every turn of the DNA double helix. Since the SV40 chromosome has 5,253 nucleotide base pairs,[1-3] the DNA strands have a topological linking number of over 500. Most of this linkage will be removed by the swivel activity (or activities) during replication of the first 95% of the SV40 chromosome. However, there are special problems at the termination of DNA replication. A "nicking-closing" activity

The SV40 Replicon Model for Analysis of Anticancer Drugs,
edited by Robert M. Snapka. ©1996 R.G. Landes Company.

such as topoisomerase I can only reduce the parental DNA strand linkage by acting on the unreplicated region of the viral genome.[4] If the swivel enzyme diffuses on and off of the unreplicated region, it will become less efficient as replication progresses, because its "target" unreplicated region will become progressively smaller. It has been suggested that this can account for the well known progressive slowing of SV40 DNA replication as it nears completion.[5] When the unreplicated region is reduced to a few turns of the helix, there may well be very little room for such an enzyme to bind and act. Molecular crowding may obscure the terminus region as the multiprotein DNA replication complexes approach one another.[6] The SV40 terminus region may also be obscured by chromatin structure. It is a region of bent DNA where a super-stable nucleosome is preferentially located.[7,8]

One solution to the termination problem would be for replication forks to stop short of complete replication of the chromosome. This would leave single stranded gaps in the terminus region. Topological linkage of the daughter chromosomes could be removed at this stage by topoisomerase I which can decatenate DNA circles containing single strand gaps.[9-11] The gaps might then be filled in by a gap-filling or "repair type" DNA synthesis. SV40 form II DNA with 22-73 nucleotide gaps in the terminus region has been reported to be a precursor to newly replicated form I molecules.[12,13]

If SV40 DNA replication is completed without complete reduction of the parental strand linkage, the two newly replicated circular daughter chromosomes will be "catenated" or topologically linked like two links in a chain (Fig. 4.1). The two daughter chromosomes making up a catenated dimer will be linked once for every turn of the parental DNA helix that was replicated without reduction of parental DNA strand linkage. Electron microscopy has been used to detect catenated dimers in SV40-infected cells.[14,15] Catenated viral genomes are always dimers composed of two identical DNA circles, a fact suggesting that they arise from DNA replication rather than recombination. However, it was thought that catenated SV40 dimers might be products of rare aberrant DNA replication events, rather than normal intermediates in the segregation of newly replicated daughter chromosomes.

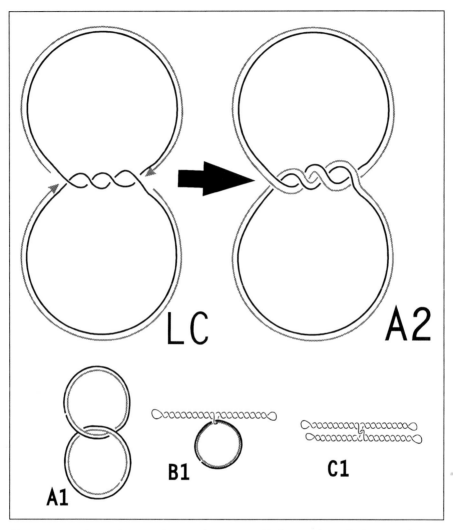

Fig. 4.1. Incomplete reduction of parental DNA strand linkage at the end of DNA replication results in catenation of the daughter chromosomes. The daughter chromosomes are linked (catenated) once for each turn of the DNA double helix that is not removed by a swivel activity during replication of the circular genome. In this diagram, two turns of the parental DNA helix are replicated without a swivel activity, converting a late Cairns replication intermediate to an A2 catenated dimer. The catenated dimer is a member of the A-family if both daughter chromosomes are relaxed due to the presence of nicks or gaps, a member of the B-family if one is relaxed and one is covalently closed, and a member of the C-family if both daughter chromosomes are covalently closed. In most cases, the covalently closed DNA circles are superhelical, however, they can be covalently closed and relaxed after in vitro digestion with topoisomerase I . There is also evidence that the covalently closed members of the B- and C-family catenated dimers may not be superhelical when the catenation linking number is very high (see text). The dimer family is indicated by the letter, and the catenation linking number is indicated by the number following the letter. The A1, B1 and C1 catenated dimers are shown.

The catenated dimers are grouped in three families based on the superhelicity of the daughter chromosomes making up each dimer. If both daughter chromosomes are relaxed due to DNA strand breaks, the dimer is a member of the A-family (Fig. 4.1, A1). If only one of the two daughter chromosomes making up a catenated dimer is superhelical, it is a member of the B-family catenated dimers (Fig 4.1, B1). Both daughter chromosomes are superhelical in a C-family catenated dimer (Fig. 4.1, C1). These catenated dimers may be singly or multiply intertwined. The number of intertwines is properly referred to as the catenation linking number (L), and is indicated by a number following the letter for the dimer family. A25 refers to a catenated dimer in which both daughter chromosomes are relaxed due to DNA strand breaks and linked to one another 25 times.

Sundin and Varshavsky provided the first good evidence that catenated dimers were normal intermediates in the segregation of newly replicated SV40 chromosomes.[6] It was suggested that late Cairns replication intermediates complete replication as A-family catenated dimers with average catenation linking numbers of 4-5, and that these are then converted first to B-family dimers as the average linking number is reduced to 2-3, then to C-family dimers with a linking number of 1-2 and finally to form I monomer DNA. They noted that decatenation could be carried out by a type II topoisomerase. Topoisomerase II changes the topology of DNA circles by a double strand DNA passing reaction in which one segment of DNA double helix is passed through a transient topoisomerase II-associated double strand gap in another segment of the DNA helix. Only topoisomerase II can knot and unknot or catenate and decatenate covalently closed double strand DNA circles.[16] Sundin and Varshavsky made extensive use of high-resolution one- and two-dimensional gel electrophoresis in their studies of catenated SV40 dimers. Each increase in catenation linking number increases the compactness of a catenated dimer. Since neutral agarose gel electrophoresis separates SV40 replication intermediates on the basis of size and compactness, the discrete increase in compactness associated with each increase in catenation linking number results in an increase in electrophoretic mobility. The A- and B-family catenated dimers thus separate into ladders of bands in one-dimensional agarose gel electrophoresis (chapter 2). Each band represents a unique catenation linking number which can be determined by band counting from the known positions of the singly catenated A-1 and B-1 dimers. The B-family dimers each contain one superhelical member, and since supercoiling also increases compactness and electrophoretic mobility on agarose gels, the B-family ladder is shifted forward relative to the A-family ladder. The A- and B-family catenated dimer ladders overlap extensively. The C-family catenated dimers with low catenation linking numbers are not resolved into a ladder by one dimensional neutral agarose gel electrophoresis but appear as a single band just behind the form II band. This may be because each increase in catenation is compensated by a decrease in the superhelicity of the daughter chromosomes.[17] In normal lytic SV40 infections, both the levels of catenated dimers and their catenation linking numbers are low. Often, the only catenated dimer bands seen are the singly catenated A1 and B1 dimer bands. However, it is not unusual to see faint B2 and B3 bands. The A2 and A3 bands tend to be obscured by the late Cairns structure on one dimensional gels. The level of catenated dimers in the normal lytic infection is a function of the multiplicity of infection,[18] thus, it is important to have untreated normal controls in any experiment involving topoisomerase II inhibition.

The first treatment discovered to inhibit the decatenation of SV40 daughter chromosomes was hypertonic shock.[19] When SV40-infected cells were treated with hypertonic media, decatenation was blocked, and highly catenated dimers (mainly C-family) accumulated at the expense of form I DNA. Since C-family (superhelical-superhelical) catenated dimers can only be separated by topoisomerase II, it was concluded that hypertonic shock must inhibit topoisomerase II and that this enzyme is responsible for separating newly replicated SV40 daughter chromosomes. This conclusion was confirmed by the observation that specific topoisomerase II inhibitors also block the decatenation step of SV40 DNA replication, causing accumulation of highly catenated dimers at the expense of form I DNA.[20,21] The idea that topoisomerase II is required for separation of newly replicated chromosomes in eukaryotic cells was strongly supported by an observation concerning the separation of newly replicated circular plasmids in yeast with a temperature sensitive topoisomerase II mutation. At the restrictive temperature, the plasmids were unable to separate and accumulated as highly catenated dimers.[22] Yeast cellular chromosomes are also unable to separate in the absence of topoisomerase II.[23-25] This indicates that cellular chromosomes, though linear, must be under similar topological constraints—possibly due to the organization of cellular chromosomes in looped domains.[26,27]

Although Sundin and Varshavsky suggested that the A-family catenated dimers might have non-complementary gaps in the terminus region,[6] this did not explain the gapped form II intermediates reported earlier to be the direct precursors of form I DNA.[12,13] A study by Weaver et al[18] reported that there are two pathways for the termination of SV40 DNA replication, one through catenated dimers and another through gapped form II DNA. This report noted that hypertonic shock slowed the completion of the late Cairns replication intermediates in addition to blocking decatenation of newly replicated daughter chromosomes—but only when replication forks meet in the normal SV40 termination region. Hypertonic shock did not slow the replication of the late Cairns structure or cause accumulation of catenated dimers when the replication forks met at other DNA sequences in altered SV40 genomes. This was interpreted to mean that the SV40 termination region favors a segregation pathway through catenated dimers when topoisomerase II activity is limited. Weaver et al[18] argued that termination occurs mainly through gapped form II molecules (without catenation) under normal physiological conditions.

As discussed in chapter 3, it is likely that topoisomerase I is the swivel activity for replication of most of the SV40 genome. The rapid breakage of DNA replication forks in the presence of the topoisomerase I poison camptothecin suggests that topoisomerase I acts on the unreplicated region at or just ahead of the DNA replication forks.[28,29] Topoisomerase II inhibition does not slow the replication of early and intermediate Cairns structures as would be expected if this enzyme were providing a significant part of the swivel activity at this stage of replication. However, specific inhibitors of topoisomerase II do slow the completion of late Cairns structures in which the terminus region remains unreplicated. Like hypertonic shock, topoisomerase II poisons such as m-AMSA (4'-[9-acridinylamino]methanesulfon-*m*-aniside), doxorubicin, Ellipticine and VM-26 slow both decatenation and completion of late Cairns replication intermediates.[20] Strong catalytic inhibitors of topoisomerase II such as 9-aminoacridine[20] and quino-benoxazines[30] slow completion of the late Cairns structure and block decatenation completely.

A "swivel switching" model for topoisomerase usage in SV40 DNA replication was proposed in 1988 to explain the simultaneous inhibition of decatenation and terminus region replication by topoisomerase II inhibitors.[20] In the swivel switching model (Fig. 4.2), topoisomerase I is the swivel activity for replication of most of the SV40 chromosome but is unable to serve this function during replication of the terminus region. In the absence of topoisomerase I activity, the replication forks continue to move, but without a swivel activity to reduce the linkage of the parental DNA strands. Movement of replication forks without a swivel activity results in intertwining of the newly replicated daughter strands. This type of intertwining provides nodes which are recognized by topoisomerase II.[31] Topoisomerase II then begins to carry out its double strand DNA passing reaction on the newly replicated daughter strands. Since topoisomerase II can reduce positive superhelical density ahead of replication forks by doing a double strand DNA passing reaction in the regions behind replication forks,[4] this action provides a swivel activity to facilitate continued replication fork movement. This model explains why catenated SV40 dimers are normally minor intermediates and why the catenation linking number is normally low. The swiveling action of topoisomerase II does not begin until replication has progressed to some extent without a swivel. From that point on, swiveling lags DNA replication—but only slightly so that decatenation is only behind by a few linkages when DNA replication is completed. These last few catenation linkages are then quickly removed by topoisomerase II which may remain associated with the catenated daughter chromosomes. Although topoisomerase II facilitates late SV40 replication by providing a swivel activity, this swivel activity is not required. Without it, late SV40 replication is slowed but not blocked. Inhibition of topoisomerase II forces DNA replication

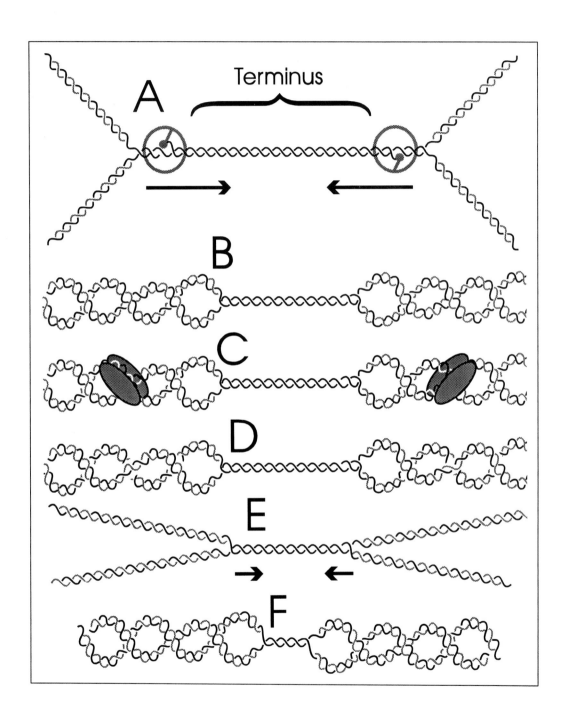

to complete without any swivel activity to reduce positive super-helical stress ahead of the replication forks, hence the dramatic slowing of DNA replication at the stage of the late Cairns structure when topoisomerase II is inhibited. The absence of a swivel activity during replication of the terminus also prevents any reduction in linkage of the parental DNA strands and produces highly catenated dimers. This model explains the close association between slowing of replication in the late Cairns structure and the level of catenation in the dimers which accumulate during inhibition of topoisomerase II.

Although hypertonic shock and a structurally diverse set of topoisomerase II inhibitors slow replication of the late Cairns structure, there are alternate explanations for this slowed replication that do not involve inhibition of topoisomerase II. For topoisomerase II poisons such as etoposide, slowed completion of the late Cairns replication intermediates might be due to physical blockage of replication forks by the drug-stabilized topoisomerase II-DNA cleavable complexes rather than to inhibition of

Fig. 4.2. (on opposite page) The swivel switching model for termination of SV40 DNA replication. This model explains the simultaneous slowing of replication in the late Cairns structure and blocking of decatenation by topoisomerase II inhibitors as well as the relationship between the level of topoisomerase II inhibition and the level of catenation in the resulting dimers. This model can accommodate all of the observations reported for the termination of SV40 DNA replication, without postulating separate pathways for segregation of daughter chromosomes. The key feature of this model is a switch from swiveling by topoisomerase I in the unreplicated region to swiveling by topoisomerase II in the replicated region as replication forks enter the terminus DNA sequences. A, topoisomerase I (solid circles) unwinds the parental DNA strands by acting on the unreplicated region ahead of the replication forks during replication of most of the SV40 genome. B, As the replication forks enter the terminus region, topoisomerase I is no longer able to act, and replication proceeds without a swivel activity to produce double strand nodes (nascent catenation) in the replicated region behind the forks. C–E, topoisomerase II (a homodimer represented by paired ellipses) recognizes these nodes and begins to unwind the parental DNA strands by carrying out a double strand DNA passing reaction behind the replication forks. This facilitates replication fork movement by reducing positive superhelical stress in the unreplicated region since the parental DNA strands are continuous through the replication forks. It also reduces the nascent catenation. F, continued replication fork movement through the terminus region generates more nascent catenation, providing new substrate for topoisomerase II. For clarity, the process is shown here as occurring in stages, but it is likely that replication of the terminus, generation of double strand nodes, and swiveling-decatenation by topoisomerase II are all occurring simultaneously. Inhibition of topoisomerase II would be expected to slow replication of the terminus region and cause catenated dimers whose catenation linking number would reflect the degree of inhibition.

topoisomerase II activity. This cannot be the case for pure catalytic inhibitors of topoisomerase II such as the quinobenoxazines since these drugs do not stabilize cleavable complexes.[30] However, these are DNA binding drugs, and DNA intercalating drugs have been reported to inhibit DNA helicases in vitro.[32] In this case, the DNA binding drugs might be slowing replication fork movement in the terminus region by interfering with helicases, DNA polymerases or other enzymes of DNA replication—and that once again slowed completion of the late Cairns structures is not due to a lack of topoisomerase II activity. Like the DNA binding drugs, hypertonic shock might inhibit other enzymes of DNA replication in addition to topoisomerase II.

Recently ICRF-193 has been reported to be a novel pre-DNA cleavage catalytic inhibitor of topoisomerase II.[33-35] This drug does not stabilize topoisomerase II–DNA cleavage complexes and is thus not a topoisomerase poison. It also does not bind to DNA. ICRF-193 binds to the free enzyme to lock it in an inactive conformation.[36] Treatment of SV40-infected cells with ICRF-193 caused blocking of SV40 decatenation and a substantial accumulation of label in the late Cairns structure band,[17] indicating that late SV40 DNA replication is slowed when topoisomerase II is inhibited. ICRF-193 also blocks replication of the SV40 terminus in an in vitro SV40 DNA replication system.[37] More recently, pulse-chase experiments were used to show that ICRF-193 does not cause a complete arrest of the SV40 replication at the stage of the late Cairns structure.[38] Since ICRF-193 does not stabilize covalent topoisomerase-DNA complexes and does not bind to DNA, it seems likely that the slowing of late SV40 replication by this drug—and other topoisomerase II inhibitors—is due to inhibition of topoisomerase II activity. This indicates that topoisomerase II facilitates late SV40 DNA replication under normal conditions.

Later work has substantiated this model. Yeast centromeric DNA sequences were reported to act as a functional replacement for the SV40 terminus region, facilitating the accumulation of late replicating intermediates and catenated dimers in SV40 under conditions of topoisomerase II depletion.[39] The authors noted that both the normal SV40 terminus region and the yeast centromeric region have A/T-rich DNA sequences which cause a bent DNA structure and suggest that bent DNA may not be a good substrate for topoisomerase II. These results were interpreted in terms of the swivel switching model discussed above.[20]

The extensive literature on termination of SV40 DNA replication can be reconciled within the framework of the swivel switching model if gap filling DNA synthesis and decatenation by topoisomerase II are concurrent processes. When there is excess topoisomerase II, removal of "nascent catenation," occurring behind replication forks approaching one another in the terminus region, occurs rapidly so that the resulting dimers have only low levels of catenation (linking numbers around 1-3). In most newly replicated molecules, the removal of the final few catenation linkages by topoisomerase II occurs very rapidly—even before the final noncomplementary single strand gaps[6] are filled. This amounts to decatenation of A1-A3 and B1-B3 dimers to produce gapped form II molecules. Filling of these single strand gaps would result in form I molecules. Thus, both catenated dimers and gapped molecules are precursors to form I and do not represent separate pathways.

Inhibition by unfavorable DNA sequences, chromatin structure, hypertonic shock or specific inhibitors causes topoisomerase II to fall behind in removing nascent catenation behind converging replication forks. This increases the level of catenation of the resulting A- and B-family catenated dimers and slows their decatenation, allowing time for gap filling DNA synthesis which converts them to covalently closed C-family dimers. The resulting C-family dimers then decatenate to give form I DNA.

Although the SV40 terminus region and other bent DNA sequences may favor the formation of catenated dimers, it is clear that topoisomerase II inhibition can cause accumulation of catenated dimers even when DNA replication forks meet in other sequences. In an in vitro SV40 DNA replication system using artificial SV40 chromosomes containing only the viral origin of DNA replication (no terminus region), depletion of topoisomerase II activity causes catenation of the daughter chromosomes.[40] Inhibition of topoisomerase II in vivo causes catenation of the SV40 circular (head-to-tail) dimer in addition to catenation of the monomeric genomes (chapter 8). In the circular dimer there are two origins of DNA replication which are 180° from one another. DNA replication forks will terminate in an origin sequence rather than a normal terminus region.

Since catenation is thought to occur during replication of the terminus region, it is likely, at least initially, to be localized to that region. This localization of catenation would facilitate decatenation by topoisomerase II in two ways: first, the region would not be obscured by chromosomal proteins; and second, topoisomerase II recognizes double strand DNA "nodes" formed by DNA helices crossing one another.[31] Evidence for localized catenation is difficult to obtain. When viral chromosomes are deproteinized, any barriers to the delocalization of catenation will be removed. Electron microscopy of catenated viral minichromosomes failed to detect any localization of catenation.[41] However, it is difficult to see DNA topology in chromatin by electron microscopy, and preparation of viral chromatin for electron microscopy requires a number of steps in which shearing and other forces might delocalize catenation. The best evidence in support of localized catenation is indirect. Two dimensional neutralchloroquine gel electrophoretic analysis of highly catenated SV40 dimers indicates that the superhelical member of the dimer becomes less superhelical as the catenation linking number increases.[17,29] This is evident in two-dimensional neutral-chloroquine gel electrophoresis of catenated SV40 dimers resulting from exposure to A-74932, a strong catalytic inhibitor of topoisomerase II (Fig. 4.3). Since the superhelicity of covalently closed SV40 DNA circles reflects the nucleosomal organization of viral chromatin (chapter 1), this suggests that there are fewer nucleosomes on highly catenated dimers. The electrophoretic behavior of C-family catenated dimers can also be interpreted in view of this idea.[17,29] If catenation is localized in the terminus region of a highly catenated dimer—as predicted by the swivel switching model—it is difficult to see how nucleosomes could be organized in the same region.

CATALYTIC TOPOISOMERASE II INHIBITORS AND TOPOISOMERASE II POISONS

Pure catalytic inhibitors of topoisomerase II inhibit topoisomerase II reactions, both in vivo and in vitro, without stabilizing the topoisomerase II reaction intermediate known as a cleavable

complex. These are sometimes known as topoisomerase II antagonists[42] since they can reduce DNA cleavage by topoisomerase II
and since they can reduce or block the enhancement of topoisomerase II-dependent DNA cleavage caused by topoisomerase II
poisons. These drugs inhibit topoisomerase II at steps preceding
(or following) DNA strand passage. The steps might be nonspecific DNA binding, consensus site recognition or DNA cleavage
itself. Some catalytic inhibitors of topoisomerase II have been shown
to have significant anticancer activity.[43,44] The antineoplastic
quinobenoxazine A-74932 is one example of a drug in this class.[30]
A-74932 reduces cleavable complexes stabilized by strong
topoisomerase poisons in vivo (Fig. 4.4). The anticancer activity
of such topoisomerase II antagonists suggests that catalytic inhibition of topoisomerase II-dependent intracellular processes is sufficient for anticancer activity. It has been widely assumed that the
anticancer activity of topoisomerase II inhibitors is due to their
activity as topoisomerase poisons which stabilize cleavable complexes.[45,46] It is clear that cleavable complexes are cytotoxic since
cells selected for resistance to these drugs often have topoisomerase
II gene mutations which reduce the stabilization of cleavable complexes by these drugs.[47-52] However, many of these same drugs inhibit topoisomerase II-dependent steps in DNA replication in vivo
as shown by their ability to cause accumulation of catenated SV40
dimers and their ability to reduce cleavable complexes stabilized
by strong topoisomerase II poisons in vivo. What are the relative
contributions of topoisomerase II poisoning and topoisomerase II
catalytic inhibition to the anticancer activity of these drugs? Is it
possible that catalytic inhibition of intracellular topoisomerase II
contributes more to selective anticancer activity, and topoisomerase
II poisoning contributes more to nonspecific toxicity to cancer cells
and normal cells? Do these factors change with different types of
tumors having different growth kinetics or different cell cycle check-
point controls? To answer these questions, a quantitative in vivo
assay for catalytic inhibition was developed to supplement the al-
ready available in vivo assays for topoisomerase poisoning. Since
inhibition of topoisomerase II causes accumulation of catenated
SV40 dimers, their levels can be taken as a measure of
topoisomerase II inhibition in vivo.

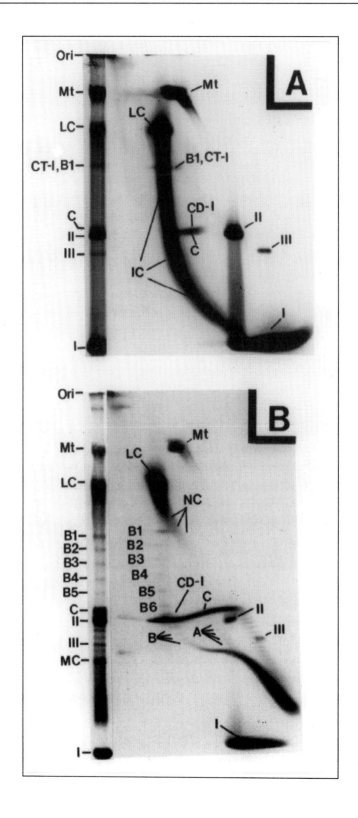

The effects of topoisomerase II inhibitors on SV40 DNA replication indicate a rough inverse relationship between topoisomerase II poisoning, as measured by drug-dependent DNA crosslinks, and topoisomerase II catalytic inhibition, as indicated by the accumulation of highly catenated dimers. This was noted in the earliest studies of the effects of topoisomerase inhibitors on SV40 DNA replication.[20] For each topoisomerase II inhibitor, there is a clear dose-response for accumulation of catenated SV40 dimers (Fig. 4.5). For the topoisomerase II poisons, there is also a clear dose-response for protein-crosslinks to SV40 DNA (chapter 2, and see Fig. 4.12 below). Topoisomerase II is the protein crosslinked to DNA in vivo by a specific topoisomerase II poison. When different topoisomerase II inhibitors are compared for levels of protein-DNA crosslinks and levels of catenated dimers at a drug concentration of 40 μM, it is clear that there are no drugs that are both strong topoisomerase II poisons and strong inhibitors of decatenation (Fig. 4.6). The Y-axis in this figure is only

Fig. 4.3. (on opposite page) Two-dimensional neutral-chloroquine gel electrophoresis of normal SV40 DNA replication intermediates (A) and intermediates caused by exposure to the quinobenoxazine topoisomerase II inhibitor A-74932 (B). Chloroquine does not alter the topology of DNA that is not covalently closed. Since A-family catenated dimers have nicks or gaps in both daughter chromosomes, their electrophoretic mobility is not significantly changed in the chloroquine second dimension electrophoresis, and the A-dimer bands make a straight diagonal in the two-dimensional pattern. Chloroquine greatly alters the electrophoretic mobility of covalently closed DNA by changing its topology. Binding of chloroquine to DNA relaxes superhelical DNA by titrating out negative supercoils.[56,57] A compact supercoiled DNA circle with high electrophoretic mobility in the first dimension electrophoretic separation thus becomes a relatively slow-migrating relaxed circle in the presence of chloroquine. However, when chloroquine binds to covalently closed relaxed DNA circles, it introduces positive supercoils, and the compact, positively supercoiled circles have a much higher electrophoretic mobility in the chloroquine second dimension than the relaxed circles had in the first dimension. Thus, chloroquine binding effectively reverses the electrophoretic mobility of covalently closed supercoiled and covalently closed relaxed DNA circles. The progressive shifting of the B-family catenated dimer bands to the right as they increase their catenation linking number indicates that the superhelical member is losing its superhelicity as a function of increasing catenation. Abbreviations: Ori, origin of electrophoresis; Mt, mitochondrial DNA; LC, late Cairns structure; B1-B5, B-family (nicked-superhelical) catenated dimers with catenation linking numbers indicated; CT-1, form I circular trimer; CD-I, form I circular dimer; C, C-family catenated dimers (unresolved); IC, intermediate Cairns structures; A, highly catenated A-family dimers; MC, pseudo-band seen in one-dimensional gel which represents the point at which B-family catenated dimers are no longer resolved; I, form I (superhelical) DNA; II, form II (nicked circular) DNA; III, form III (double strand linear) DNA. See chapter 2 for details of the gel system and structures of the intermediates. (Paskasari A. Permana, unpublished data).

Fig. 4.4. A-74932 is an antagonist of the topoisomerase II poison VM-26 but not the topoisomerase I poison camptothecin. A, Topoisomerase I-SV40 DNA complexes stabilized by 40 µM camptothecin were not affected by pretreatment with the antineoplastic quinobenoxazine A-74932. B, Protein-DNA crosslinks caused by 100 µM VM-26 were reduced in a dose-dependent manner by exposure to A-74932. SV40 infected CV-1 cells were labeled with tritiated thymidine for 30 min. A-74932 was added for the last 20 min of labeling, and the topoisomerase poisons were added for the last 15 min of labeling. At the end of the labeling and drug exposure, the media containing label and drugs was removed and replaced with Hirt lysing fluid (chapter 2). Samples were taken directly from Hirt extract supernatants of drug-treated SV40-infected cells and assayed for protein-DNA crosslinks by the GF/C filter assay (chapter 2). Only SV40 chromosomes covalently crosslinked to topoisomerase I or topoisomerase II are bound to the filter in 0.4 M guanidinium chloride. In 4.0 M guanidinium chloride, all SV40 DNA binds to the filter (maximum bind-

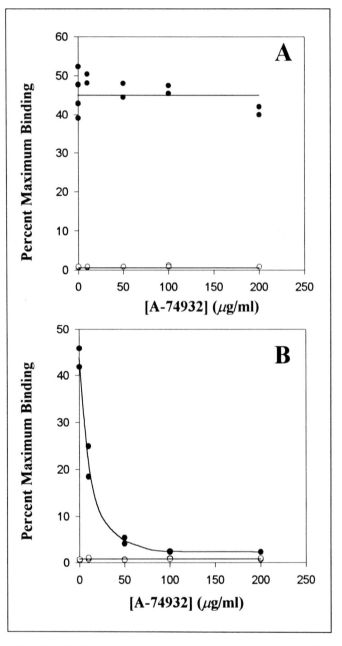

ing). The percentage of labeled SV40 DNA crosslinked to a topoisomerase is expressed as "percent maximum binding." Duplicate samples were assayed after digestion with proteinase K to demonstrate that the filter binding was due to protein-DNA crosslinks. (Paskasari A. Permana, unpublished data).

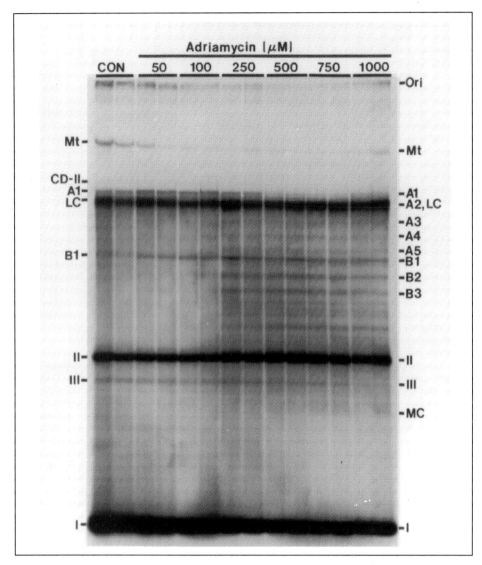

Fig. 4.5. Adriamycin dose-response for accumulation of catenated SV40 dimers. SV40-infected CV-1 cells were pulse-labeled with tritiated thymidine (250 µCi/ml) for 30 min, with increasing concentrations of Adriamycin being present in the last 15 min of the labeling. Labeling solution was replaced by Hirt lysis fluid, and viral DNA was prepared for electrophoresis by deproteinization of the Hirt extract supernatant, ethanol precipitation, and resuspension in gel loading buffer. One-dimensional neutral agarose gel electrophoresis (chapter 2) was carried out on the samples, and bands representing pulse-labeled SV40 DNA replication intermediates were visualized by gel fluorography. Abbreviations: Con, control (solvent); Ori, origin of electrophoresis; Mt, mitochondrial DNA; I, Form I (superhelical) SV40 DNA; II, form II (nicked circular DNA); III, form III (double strand linear DNA); CD-II, form II circular (head-to-tail dimer); LC, late Cairns replication intermediate; A1-n, A-family catenated dimers with catenation linkage indicated; B1-n, B-family catenated dimers; MC, pseudo-band at the point where B-family catenated dimer bands are no longer resolved. (Christopher A. Ferrer, unpublished data).

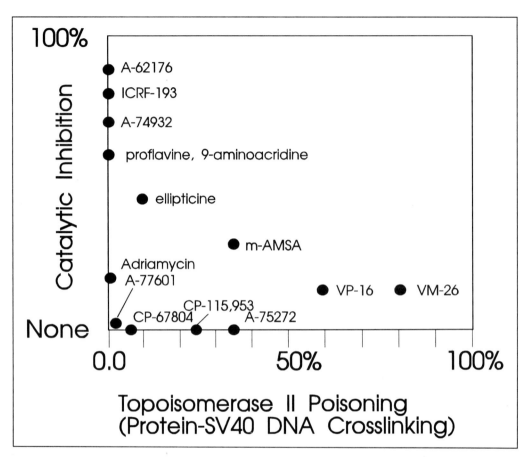

Fig. 4.6. Topoisomerase II poisoning and catalytic inhibition of topoisomerase II in vivo. A variety of topoisomerase II inhibitors were compared for their effects on SV40 DNA replication intermediates when added to virus-infected cells for 15 min at a concentration of 40 μM. Topoisomerase II poisoning was measured as protein crosslinks to pulse-labeled SV40 DNA as measured with the GF/C filter assay (chapter 2). The samples were also analyzed by one-dimensional agarose gel electrophoresis. Levels of catenated dimers are taken as a measure of catalytic inhibition of topoisomerase II. The levels of catenated dimers were estimated based on band intensities relative to other intermediates in identical fluorographic exposures. The drugs were then ranked for the levels of catenated dimers between zero (no drug treatment) and 100% (hypertonic shock). Drugs located precisely on the Y-axis do not cause detectable protein-DNA crosslinks and are not topoisomerase II poisons. For drugs located precisely on the X-axis, catenated SV40 dimers are not detected. A-62176, A-74932, A-77601 and A-75272 were gifts of Abbott Laboratories. VP-16 (etoposide), VM-26 (teniposide), and m-AMSA (4'-[9-acridinyl-amino]-methanesulfon-m-aniside) were provided by the National Cancer Institute, CP-67804 and CP-115,953 were gifts of Pfizer, Inc., and ICRF-193 was a gift of Zenyaku Kogyo Co., Ltd., Tokyo. All other inhibitors were purchased from Sigma Chemical Co.

semiquantitative. For more complete studies of the disruption of DNA replication in vivo by topoisomerase II inhibitors, it was necessary to have a quantitative measure of topoisomerase II inhibition in SV40-infected cells. Since the accumulation of catenated dimers is a measure of topoisomerase II inhibition in vivo, we have developed quantitative assays for catenated dimers.

ASSAYS FOR CATENATED DIMERS

ASSAY FOR C-FAMILY CATENATED DIMERS

Although two dimensional gel electrophoresis does an excellent job of separating different SV40 DNA replication intermediates, the best separations are still inadequate for densitometric quantification of specific forms. This is especially true for the ladders of catenated dimer bands which tend to overlap or partially overlap the bands of other replication intermediates at various points in two-dimensional gel electrophoresis patterns. However, the pattern can be simplified by selectively removing intermediates that interfere with the analysis of catenated dimers. The first assay of this type to be developed was an assay for C-family catenated dimers. The rationale of the assay is shown in Figure 4.7. Purified SV40 DNA replication intermediates are briefly heat denatured at 90°C and then renatured after quenching in a dry ice/ethanol bath. Intermediates with DNA strand breaks are irreversibly denatured, and covalently closed forms are renatured by this procedure. The covalently closed forms are form I SV40 DNA and the C-family catenated dimers. The denatured intermediates, which bind to nitrocellulose, are removed by passage through a nitrocellulose filter. Mitochondrial DNA and other traces of contaminating cellular DNA are also removed by the denaturation-renaturation and filtration. A pulsed-field electrophoresis protocol is then used to separate the renatured, covalently closed SV40 intermediates which pass through the filter. Pulsed-field electrophoresis is used because a significant amount of form II DNA can arise by radiolysis of the heavily labeled form I DNA during the filtration step and preparation for electrophoresis. It is difficult to completely separate C-family catenated dimers from form II DNA by any of the one- or two-dimensional electrophoresis protocols in

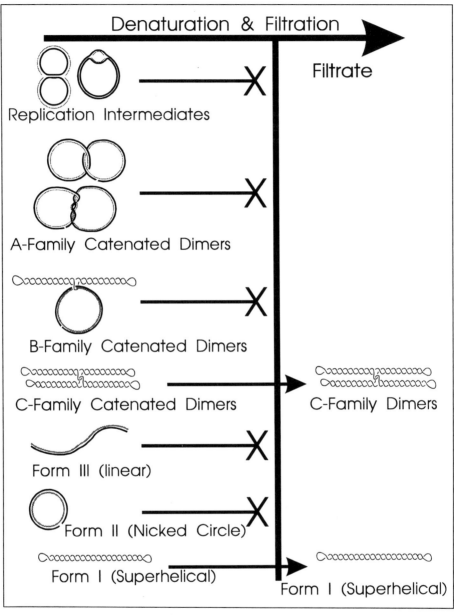

Fig. 4.7. The assay for C-family catenated dimers. Rapid heating and cooling irreversibly denatures SV40 DNA replication intermediates with single and double strand DNA breaks. The denatured intermediates are removed by passage through a nitrocellulose filter. Only covalently closed intermediates renature and pass through the filter. The viral DNA, purified from the Hirt extract supernatant, is heated at 90 °C for 5 min in TE buffer (10 mM Tris HCl, 1.0 mM EDTA, pH 7.5) and is then moved quickly to a dry ice-ethanol bath. Frozen samples (100 µl) are thawed at 4 °C, adjusted to 1.0 M NaCl, and passed through a 0.45 micron nitrocellulose filter (Alltech) that has been pre-wetted with the same buffer. The filter is rinsed three times with 125 µl aliquots of 1.0 M NaCl and the DNA in the filtrate is concentrated by ethanol precipitation.

routine use in the laboratory. However, extensive characterization of the pulsed-field separation has shown that the order of SV40 intermediates is: form III (highest electrophoretic mobility), form I, form II, catenated dimers (A-, B- and C-families). When SV40 replication intermediates from cells treated with the catalytic topoisomerase II inhibitors ICRF-193 and A-62176 were analyzed with this assay, a clear dose-response was obtained for the formation of catenated dimers (Fig. 4.8). Other experiments with two-dimensional gels confirmed that forms I, II and catenated dimers are the only intermediates present in these samples. Topoisomerase II poisons also cause measurable accumulation of C-family catenated dimers in this assay, although at significantly lower levels than those caused by strong topoisomerase II antagonists like ICRF-193 and A-62176 (Fig. 4.9). There is a linear relationship between densitometric peak area and fluorographic exposure time for bands of tritium-labeled SV40 intermediates in agarose gels. By making several exposures, slopes can be obtained for each band (Fig. 4.10). The ratio of slope for the catenated dimer area and slopes for the form I and II bands gives the ratio of C-family catenated dimers to form I DNA at the time of filtration. The C-dimer/form I ratio from untreated control cells is set to one, and the levels of SV40 dimers in the treated cells are normalized to the untreated cells. Since inhibition of SV40 decatenation causes an accumulation of pulse-label in catenated dimers at the expense of form I DNA, the ratio of C-family dimers to form I DNA is a sensitive function of topoisomerase II inhibition. Normalized C-family catenated dimers can then be plotted as a function of drug dose (Fig. 4.11). The data from an assay for catenated dimers can be plotted with the drug concentration and the drug-induced protein-DNA crosslinks on a three axis graph (Fig. 4.12). Each concentration of drug causes specific levels of catenated dimers, and protein-DNA crosslinks. Thus, the data can be plotted to show protein-DNA crosslinks as a function of C-family catenated dimers (Fig. 4.13). For the DNA intercalating topoisomerase II poisons m-AMSA and Ellipticine, there is a steep increase in topoisomerase poisoning followed by a plateau where cleavable complexes do not change significantly with increasing accumulation of C-family catenated dimers. Ellipticine is the weaker of the two topoisomerase II poisons.

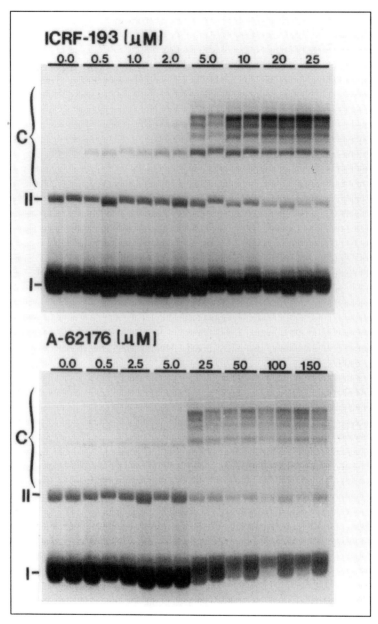

Fig. 4.8. Pulsed-field gel electrophoresis of C-family catenated SV40 dimers: dose-response for the topoisomerase II antagonists ICRF-193 and A-62176. I, form I (superhelical) SV40 DNA; II, form II (nicked circle); C, C-family catenated dimers. Viral DNA extracted from tritium pulse-labeled drug-treated cells was prepared by denaturation/renaturation and nitrocellulose filtration (Fig. 4.7). The ethanol precipitated DNA pellet was dried briefly, then taken up in gel loading buffer. Pulsed field gel electrophoresis (24 hr; 4 V/cm, 0.5 sec forward/ null 0.2 sec) was done in a 1% agarose gel in 0.25X TBE buffer (1X TBE = 89 mM Tris, 89 mM borate, 2 mM EDTA) using a Hoefer PC750 pulse controller. The gel was processed for fluorography (chapter 2) and exposed to Kodak X-Omat AR film at -80°C.

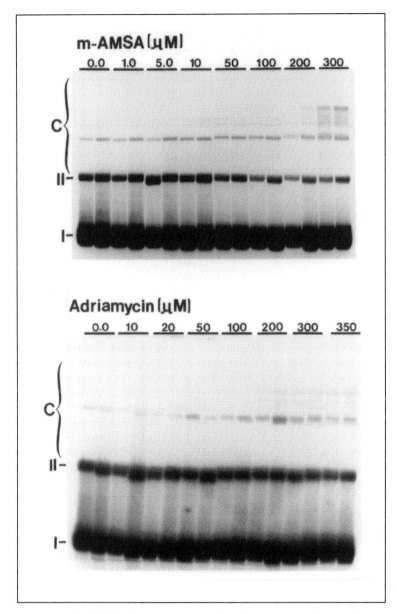

Fig. 4.9. Pulsed-field gel electrophoresis of C-family catenated SV40 dimers: dose-response for the DNA binding topoisomerase II poisons m-AMSA and Adriamycin. Abbreviations, preparation of DNA and electrophoresis details are given in Figure 4.8.

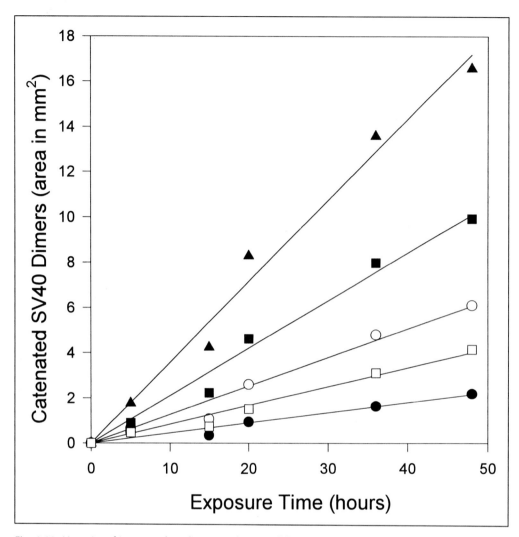

Fig. 4.10. Linearity of integrated peak area with time of fluorographic exposure for C-family catenated dimers measured by soft laser densitometry. Proflavine was added to SV40 infected cells during a pulse-labeling with tritiated thymidine, and the assay for C-family catenated dimers was carried out as shown in Figs. 4.7-4.9. A series of fluorographic exposures were made for times ranging from 5 to 48 hr. The region of C-family catenated SV40 dimers was scanned with a soft laser densitometer (LKB) in each fluorograph. A plot of integrated peak area versus time of exposure for each drug concentration gives a straight line whose slope is proportional to the level of C-family catenated dimers in the sample. The increasing slopes give a quantitative measure of catalytic inhibition of topoisomerase II in vivo by proflavine. ●, no drug; ❑, 12 μM proflavine; ○, 15 μM proflavine; ■, 20 μM proflavine; ▲, 30 μM proflavine.

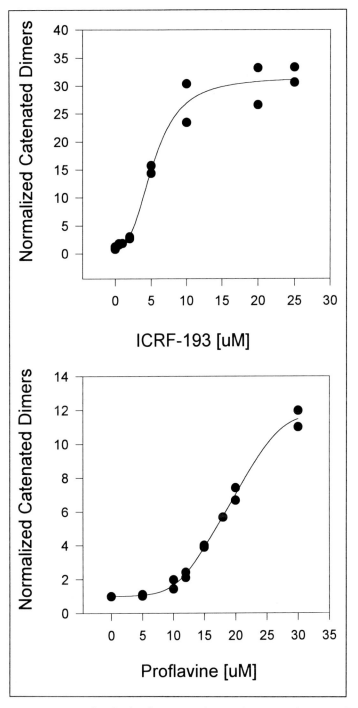

Fig. 4.11. Normalized C-family catenated SV40 dimers as a function of
drug dose for ICRF-193 and proflavine.

When the data for normalized C-family catenated dimers are plotted against drug dose for a variety of topoisomerase II inhibitors, the pure catalytic topoisomerase II inhibitors (ICRF-193, A-62176, A-74932 and proflavine) are clearly separated from the topoisomerase II poisons (Adriamycin, m-AMSA and VP-16) (Fig. 4.14). Ellipticine is intermediate. This separation is probably due to topoisomerase II poisons stabilizing cleavable complexes on the catenated dimers. This is known to be the case for several of

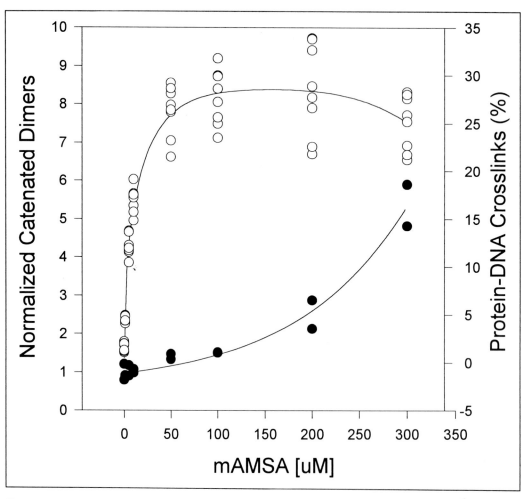

Fig. 4.12. Protein-DNA crosslinks and normalized C-family catenated SV40 dimers as a function of m-AMSA dose. ○, protein-DNA crosslinks; ●, normalized C-family catenated dimers. The protein-DNA crosslink is a measure of topoisomerase II poisoning activity and is taken from four experiments done over a four month period. The normalized catenated dimer data was taken from two of those experiments.

the topoisomerase II poisons.[53] Since the cleavable complex is a protein associated DNA strand break, a significant fraction of the catenated dimers caused by topoisomerase II poisons will be A-, and B-family catenated dimers which are removed by this assay. The DNA intercalating topoisomerase II poisons (m-AMSA and Adriamycin) cause accumulation of C-family catenated dimers only at very high drug concentrations. These drugs are known to cause

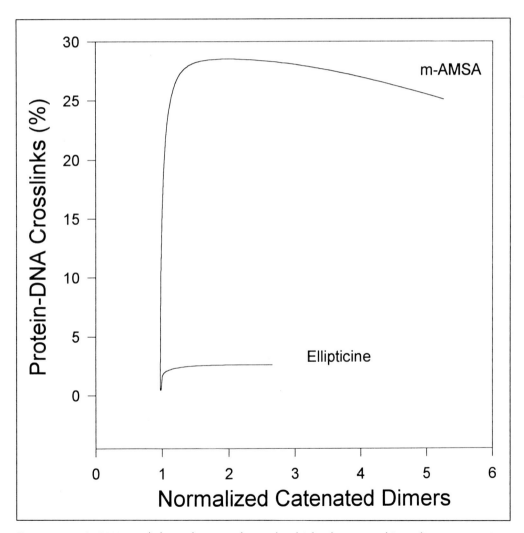

Fig. 4.13. Protein-DNA crosslinks as a function of normalized C-family catenated SV40 dimers: comparison of Ellipticine and m-AMSA. The m-AMSA data from Figure 4.12 was re-plotted to show protein-DNA crosslinks as a function of normalized C-family catenated dimers. Similar data for Ellipticine was added for comparison.

"self-inhibition" of their own topoisomerase II poisoning at high concentrations.[54] In this case, C-family catenated dimers apparently only accumulate when the drug concentration is high enough to interfere with its own ability to stabilize cleavable complexes. There is also a difference between the non-DNA binding topoisomerase II

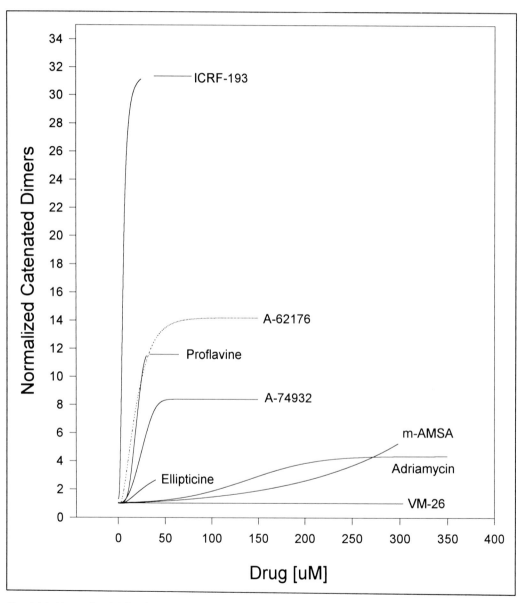

Fig. 4.14. *Normalized C-family catenated dimers as a function of drug dose for several topoisomerase II antagonists and topoisomerase II poisons.*

antagonist ICRF-193 and the DNA binding quinobenoxazines A-62176 and A-74932. ICRF-193 appears to be a much stronger inducer of C-family catenated dimers. This does not necessarily mean that A-62176 and A-74932 are weaker topoisomerase II antagonists. As DNA binding drugs, they may interfere with ligation of Okazaki fragments or with gap filling in the late stage of SV40 DNA replication. One dimensional agarose gel electrophoresis of unfractionated SV40 DNA replication intermediates suggests that A-62176 and ICRF-193 cause comparable levels of catenated dimers, but C-family dimers predominate with ICRF-193. A different assay is thus required to obtain a measure of total catenated dimers and a quantitative estimate of topoisomerase II catalytic inhibition.

ASSAY FOR TOTAL CATENATED DIMERS

The quantitative assay for total catenated SV40 dimers involves dividing the purified SV40 DNA from each sample into two aliquots. One aliquot is digested with DNase I in the presence of ethidium bromide to convert all superhelical forms to nicked forms. Relaxation of superhelical DNA by DNase I nicking allows it to take up much more of the ethidium bromide, which inhibits more nicking by the enzyme.[55] This treatment converts form I DNA to form II and B- and C-family catenated dimers to A-family catenated dimers. One-dimensional pulsed-field electrophoresis of the DNase I-digested sample gives a simple pattern consisting of a form III band followed by an intense form II band. All of the A-family catenated dimers and nicked Cairns replication intermediates produced by DNase I nicking are located in the region behind the form II band. Densitometric scanning of this region gives a value for catenated dimers plus Cairns replication intermediates. This value can be expressed as a fraction of total labeled SV40 DNA.

The other aliquot is digested to completion with the restriction endonuclease Bgl I which cuts SV40 DNA once near the origin of DNA replication (Fig. 4.15). In the Bgl I digestion, forms I and II and the catenated dimers are converted to form III DNA while the pre-existing form III DNA is reduced to smaller fragments. Cairns replication intermediates are converted to X-forms as shown. One-dimensional pulsed field agarose gel electrophoresis

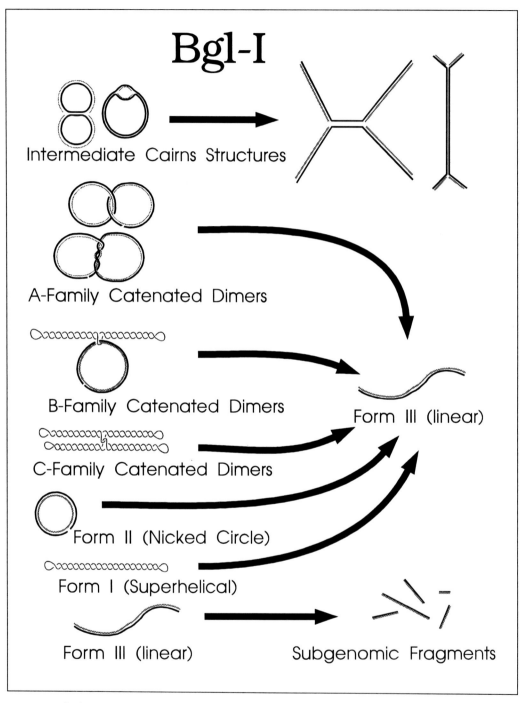

Fig. 4.15. Bgl I digestion of SV40 DNA replication intermediates. Intermediate Cairns structures are converted to X-forms while all other intermediates are converted to form III DNA or to subgenomic fragments.

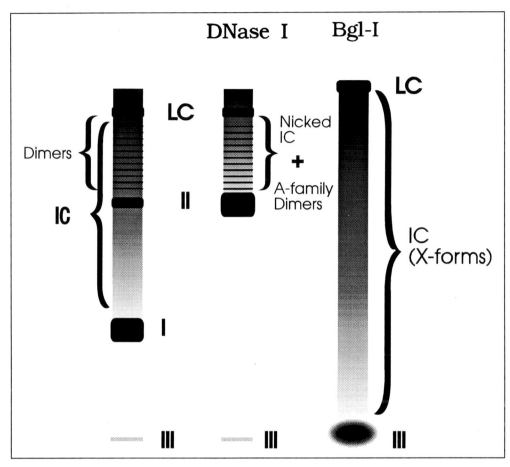

Fig. 4.16. Assay of total catenated SV40 dimers by pulsed-field agarose gel electrophoresis of DNase I and Bgl I digested SV40 DNA replication intermediates. The left lane shows the pattern of SV40 intermediates separated by pulsed-field agarose gel electrophoresis. The A-, B-, and C-family catenated dimers are all found in the region between the form II band and the late Cairns structure (LC). Intermediate Cairns structures (IC) are distributed as a continuous smear from the form I band to the late Cairns band. To assay total catenated dimers, the sample is divided into two aliquots, and one is subjected to controlled DNase I nicking while the other is digested to completion with Bgl I. Controlled DNase I nicking converts all three families of catenated SV40 dimers to A-family dimers, form I DNA to form II, and intermediate Cairns structures to nicked intermediate Cairns structures. The resulting nicked intermediate Cairns structures and A-family dimers are distributed between the form II DNA band and the late Cairns structure after separation by pulsed-field electrophoresis. In the pulsed-field electrophoresis pattern of Bgl I-digested SV40 intermediates, the X-form intermediate Cairns structures are distributed in the region behind the form III band. All other intermediates have been converted to form III or smaller fragments by the Bgl I digestion. Intermediate Cairns structures can be quantitated by densitometry of this region. This value is subtracted from the value for nicked intermediate Cairns structures and A-family dimers obtained by densitometry of the DNase I digest to obtain a value for total catenated SV40 dimers in the sample.

of the Bgl I digest gives a very simple pattern consisting of an intense band of form III DNA followed by a smear of X-form replication intermediates (Fig. 4.16). This allows densitometric quantitation of the intermediate Cairns structures as a fraction of total labeled SV40 DNA. The DNase I digest gives a value for total catenated dimers plus Cairns replication intermediates. The Bgl I digest gives a value for Cairns replication intermediates, and the value for total catenated dimers can be obtained by subtraction.

REFERENCES

1. Reddy VB, Thimmappaya B, Dhar R et al. The genome of simian virus 40. Science 1978; 200:494-502.
2. Fiers W, Contreras R, Haegemann G et al. Complete nucleotide sequence of SV40 DNA. Nature 1978; 273:113-120.
3. Tooze J. DNA tumor viruses. Cold Spring Harbor Laboratory, 1991.
4. Been MD, Champoux JJ. Topoisomerases and the swivel problem. In: Alberts B, Fox CF, eds. Mechanistic Studies of DNA Replication and Genetic Recombination. New York: Academic Press, Inc. 1980:809-15.
5. Levine AJ, Van der Vliet PC, Sussenbach JS. The replication of papovavirus and adenovirus DNA. Current Topics in Microbiology and Immunology 1976; 73:67-124.
6. Sundin O, Varshavsky A. Terminal stages of SV40 DNA replication proceed via multiply intertwined catenated dimers. Cell 1980; 21:103-114.
7. Poljak LG, Gralla JD. Competition for formation of nucleosomes on fragmented SV40 DNA: a hyperstable nucleosome forms on the terminus region. Biochemistry 1987; 26:295-303.
8. Hsieh C-H, Griffith JD. The terminus of SV40 DNA replication and transcription contains a sharp sequence-directed curve. Cell 1988; 52:535-544.
9. Holden JA, Low RL. Characterization of a potent catenation activity of HeLa cell nuclei. J Biol Chem 1985; 260:14491-14497.
10. McCoubrey WK, Champoux JJ. The role of single-strand breaks in the catenation reaction catalyzed by the rat type I topoisomerase. J Biol Chem 1986; 261:5130-5137.
11. Brown PO, Cozzarelli NR. Catenation and knotting of duplex DNA by type 1 topoisomerases: a mechanistic parallel with type 2 topoisomerases. Proc Natl Acad Sci USA 1981; 78:843-847.
12. Tapper DP, Anderson S, DePamphilis M. Distribution of replicating simian virus 40 DNA in intact cells and its maturation in isolated nuclei. J Virol 1982; 41:877-892.

13. Chen MCY, Birkenmeier E, Salzman NP. Simian virus 40 DNA replication: characterization of gaps in the termination region. J Virol 1976; 17:614-621.

14. Rush MG, Eason R, Vinograd J. Identification and properties of complex forms of SV40 DNA isolated from SV40-infected african green monkey (BSC-I) cells. Biochim Biophys Acta 1970; 228:585-594.

15. Jaenisch R, Levine A. DNA replication in SV40-infected cells. V. Circular and catenated oligomers of SV40 DNA. Virology 1971; 44:480-493.

16. Wang JC. DNA topoisomerases. Ann Rev Biochem 1985; 54:665-697.

17. Permana PA, Ferrer CA, Snapka RM. Inverse relationship between catenation and superhelicity in newly replicated simian virus 40 daughter chromosomes. Biochem Biophys Res Commun 1994; 201:1510-1517.

18. Weaver DT, Fields-Berry SC, DePamphilis ML. The termination region for SV40 DNA replication directs the mode of separation for the two sibling molecules. Cell 1985; 41:565-575.

19. Sundin O, Varshavsky A. Arrest of segregation leads to accumulation of highly intertwined catenated dimers: dissection of the final stages of SV40 DNA replication. Cell 1981; 25:659-669.

20. Snapka RM, Powelson MA, Strayer JM. Swiveling and decatenation of replicating simian virus 40 genomes in vivo. Mol Cell Biol 1988; 8:515-521.

21. Snapka RM. Topoisomerase inhibitors can selectively interfere with different stages of simian virus 40 DNA replication. Mol Cell Biol 1986; 6:4221-4227.

22. DiNardo S, Voekel K, Sternglanz R. DNA topoisomerase II mutant of *Saccharomyces cerevisiae*: topoisomerase II is required for segregation of daughter molecules at the termination of DNA replication. Proc Natl Acad Sci USA 1984; 81:2616-2620.

23. Yanagida M. Gene products required for chromosome separation. J Cell Sci 1989; 94 Suppl. 12:213-229.

24. Holm C, Stearns T, Botstein D. DNA topoisomerase II must act at mitosis to prevent nondisjunction and chromosome breakage. Mol Cell Biol 1989; 9:159-168.

25. Uemura T, Yanagida M. Mitotic spindle pulls but fails to separate chromosomes in type II DNA topoisomerase mutants: uncoordinated mitosis. EMBO J 1986; 5:1003-1010.

26. Jackson DA, Dickinson P, Cook PR. The size of chromatin loops in HeLa cells. EMBO J 1990; 9:567-571.

27. Schleif R. DNA looping. Ann Rev Biochem 1992; 61:199-223.

28. Shin C-G, Snapka RM. Exposure to camptothecin breaks leading

and lagging strand simian virus 40 DNA replication forks. Biochem Biophys Res Commun 1990; 168:135-140.

29. Snapka RM, Permana PA. SV40 DNA replication intermediates: analysis of drugs which target mammalian DNA replication. BioEssays 1993; 15:121-127.

30. Permana PA, Snapka RM, Shen LL et al. Quinobenoxazines: A class of novel antitumor quinolones and potent mammalian DNA topoisomerase II catalytic inhibitors. Biochemistry 1994; 33: 11333-11339.

31. Zechiedrich EL, Osheroff N. Eukaryotic topoisomerases recognize nucleic acid topology by preferentially interacting with DNA cross-overs. EMBO J 1990; 9:4555-4562.

32. Bachur NR, Yu F, Johnson R et al. Helicase inhibition by anthracycline anticancer agents. Mol Pharmacol 1992; 41:993-998.

33. Ishida R, Hamatake M, Wasserman RA et al. DNA topoisomerase II is the molecular target of bisdioxopiperazine derivatives ICRF-159 and ICRF-193 in *Saccharomyces cerevisiae*. Cancer Res 1995; 55:2299-2303.

34. Tanabe K, Ikegami Y, Ishida R et al. Inhibition of topoisomerase II by antitumor agents bis(2,6-dioxopiperazine) derivatives. Cancer Res 1991; 51:4903-4908.

35. Ishida R, Miki T, Narita T et al. Inhibition of intracellular topoisomerase II by antitumor bis(2,6-dioxopiperazine) derivatives: mode of cell growth inhibition distinct from that of cleavable complex-forming type inhibitors. Cancer Res 1991; 51:4909-4916.

36. Roca J, Ishida R, Berger JM et al. Antitumor bisdioxopiperazines inhibit yeast DNA topoisomerase II by trapping the enzyme in the form of a closed protein clamp. Proc Natl Acad Sci USA 1994; 91:1781-1785.

37. Ishimi Y, Ishida R, Andoh T. Effect of ICRF-193, a novel DNA topoisomerase II inhibitor, on simian virus 40 DNA and chromosome replication in vitro. Mol Cell Biol 1992; 12:4007-4014.

38. Ishimi Y, Ishida R, Andoh T. Synthesis of simian virus 40 C-family catenated dimers in vivo in the presence of ICRF-193. J Mol Biol 1995; 247:835-839.

39. Fields-Berry SC, DePamphilis ML. Sequences that promote formation of catenated intertwines during termination of DNA replication. Nucleic Acids Res 1989; 17:3261-3274.

40. Yang L, Wold MS, Li JJ et al. Roles of DNA topoisomerases in simian virus 40 DNA replication in vitro. Proc Natl Acad Sci USA 1987; 84:950-954.

41. Varshavsky A, Sundin O, Ozkaynak E, et al. Final stages of DNA replication: multiply intertwined catenated dimers as SV40 segregation intermediates. In: Cozzarelli NR, ed. Mechanisms of DNA

Replication and Recombination. New York: Alan R. Liss, 1983:463-94.

42. Shin C-G, Strayer JM, Wani MA et al. Rapid evaluation of topoisomerase inhibitors: caffeine inhibition of topoisomerases in vivo. Teratogen Carcinogen Mutagen 1990; 10:41-52.

43. Chu DTW, Hallas R, Clement JJ et al. Synthesis and antitumor activities of quinolone antineoplastic agents. Drugs Exptl Clin Res 1992; 18:275-282.

44. Ishida R, Sato M, Narita T et al. Inhibition of DNA topoisomerase II by ICRF-193 induces polyploidization by uncoupling chromosome dynamics from other cell cycle events. J Cell Biol 1994; 126:1341-1351.

45. D'Arpa P, Liu LF. Topoisomerase-targeting antitumor drugs. Biochim Biophys Acta 1989; 989:163-177.

46. Liu LF. DNA topoisomerase poisons as antitumor drugs. Ann Rev Biochem 1989; 58:351-75.

47. Zwelling LA, Bales E, Altschuler E et al. Circumvention of resistance by doxorubicin, but not by idarubicin, in a human leukemia cell line containing an intercalator-resistant form of topoisomerase II: Evidence for a non-topoisomerase II-mediated mechanism of doxorubicin cytotoxicity. Biochem Pharmacol 1993; 45:516-520.

48. Zwelling LA, Hinds M, Chan D et al. Characterization of an amsacrine-resistant line of human leukemia cells. Evidence for a drug-resistant form of topoisomerase II. J Biol Chem 1989; 264:16411-16420.

49. Chen M, Beck WT. Teniposide-resistant CEM cells, which express mutant DNA topoisomerase IIα, when treated with non-complex-stabilizing inhibitors of the enzyme, display no cross-resistance and reveal aberrant functions of the mutant enzyme. Cancer Res 1993; 53:5946-5953.

50. Mirski SEL, Evans CD, Almquist KC et al. Altered topoisomerase IIα in a drug-resistant small cell lung cancer cell line selected in VP-16. Cancer Res 1993; 53:4866-4873.

51. Bugg BY, Danks MK, Beck WT et al. Expression of a mutant DNA topoisomerase II in CCRF-CEM human leukemic cells selected for resistance to teniposide. Proc Natl Acad Sci USA 1991; 88: 7654-7658.

52. Boege F, Biersack H, Meyer P. Drug-sensitivity and DNA-binding of a subform of topoisomerase IIα in resistant human HL-60 cells. Acta Oncol 1994; 33:799-806.

53. Shin C-G, Snapka RM. Patterns of strongly protein-associated simian virus 40 DNA replication intermediates resulting from exposures to specific topoisomerase poisons. Biochemistry 1990; 29:10934-10939.

54. Crow RT, Crothers DM. Inhibition of topoisomerase I by anthracycline antibiotics: evidence for general inhibition of topoisomerase I by DNA-binding drugs. J Med Chem 1994; 16:3191-3194.

55. Greenfield L, Simpson L, Kaplan D. Conversion of closed circular DNA molecules to single-nicked molecules by digestion with DNAase I in the presence of ethidium bromide. Biochim Biophys Acta 1975; 407:365-375.

56. Bauer W, Vinograd J. Circular DNA. In: Ts'o POP, ed. Basic Principles in Nucleic Acid Chemistry. New York: Academic Press, Inc. 1974:265-303.

57. Shure M, Pulleyblank DE, Vinograd J. The problems of eukaryotic and prokaryotic DNA packaging and in vivo conformation posed by superhelix heterogeneity. Nucleic Acids Res 1977; 4:1183-1205.

========= CHAPTER 5 =========

DNA DAMAGING AGENTS

Robert M. Snapka

DNA replication can be disrupted by DNA damage as well as inhibition of DNA replication enzymes. DNA damaging agents make up an important class of anticancer drugs that includes DNA nicking agents such as bleomycin, DNA alkylating agents and DNA crosslinking agents. Ionizing radiation, one of the most useful anticancer treatments, targets DNA. DNA damaging agents are also mutagenic and carcinogenic. A great deal is known about the DNA lesions caused by different DNA damaging agents, and the enzymology of DNA repair is a mature, rapidly advancing field. Programmed cell death in response to DNA damage is a younger field, but is developing rapidly. The interactions of specific DNA lesions with cellular enzymes of DNA replication and transcription are not well understood. There is good evidence that cell killing by camptothecin is mediated by collisions of DNA replication forks with drug-stabilized topoisomerase I-DNA cleavage complexes (chapter 3). The lethal lesion is not the drug-stabilized cleavable complex but the broken DNA replication fork resulting from the collision. SV40 was the system used to discover this collision and replication fork breakage.[1] A substantial amount of work with camptothecin toxicity and double strand breaks in mammalian cells is consistent with the SV40-derived model for the toxic lesion. Because of the difficulty of working with mammalian chromosomes, however, much of the evidence supporting the presence of this lesion in cellular chromosomes after camptothecin exposure remains

The SV40 Replicon Model for Analysis of Anticancer Drugs,
edited by Robert M. Snapka. ©1996 R.G. Landes Company.

indirect and suggestive. Only a simplified system such as SV40 can provide the molecular detail of events such as replication fork collisions with DNA lesions. To help fill the information gap between DNA damage and cell death, we need to understand how the damage affects DNA replication and transcription at the molecular level. This information will be important for both carcinogenesis and cancer chemotherapy.

REACTIVE ALDEHYDES

Aldehydes are a class of reactive compounds that make covalent adducts to a variety of cellular macromolecules, including DNA. They are ubiquitous pollutants produced by many types of combustion such as smoking, operation of diesel powered engines, and fires used for cooking and heating.[2,3] A number of aldehydes are bifunctional and capable of crosslinking proteins to DNA or to one another.[4] Formaldehyde is the most extensively studied member of this class of genotoxins. In addition to being produced by combustion, it is emitted by cleaning agents, home furnishings and construction materials.[2,3] High levels of formaldehyde exposure are associated with some industrial processes.[3] Formaldehyde is an efficient protein-DNA crosslinker,[4] and it is a mutagen in mice, human cells, *Drosophila*, bacteria and fungi.[2] Formaldehyde is a potent clastogen capable of causing a variety of chromosomal rearrangements, and it is carcinogenic to rodents when supplied in drinking water or air.[5] Formaldehyde is also a normal cellular metabolite.[2,3]

The three bifunctional aldehydes, formaldehyde, acrolein and glutaraldehyde (Fig. 5.1), are known to be very efficient protein-DNA crosslinkers, whereas monofunctional aldehydes such as acetaldehyde, propionaldehyde, glyoxal, benzaldehyde and furfural cause very few protein-DNA crosslinks.[4] To understand how aldehyde-induced protein-DNA crosslinks affect DNA replication in mammalian cells, a variety of reactive aldehydes were studied for their effects on SV40 DNA replication.[6] The three bifunctional aldehydes showed a strong dose-response for protein crosslinks to replicating SV40 chromosomes. The monofunctional agents did not cause detectable protein-SV40 DNA crosslinks. SV40 DNA replication was unaffected by high concentrations of the

monofunctional aldehydes, but the bifunctional aldehydes caused
40S intermediates. This shows that protein-DNA crosslinks cause
40S intermediates in replicating SV40 genomes. This accumulation of 40S intermediates is relatively weak compared to that caused
by the DNA polymerase inhibitor aphidicolin (chapter 3).

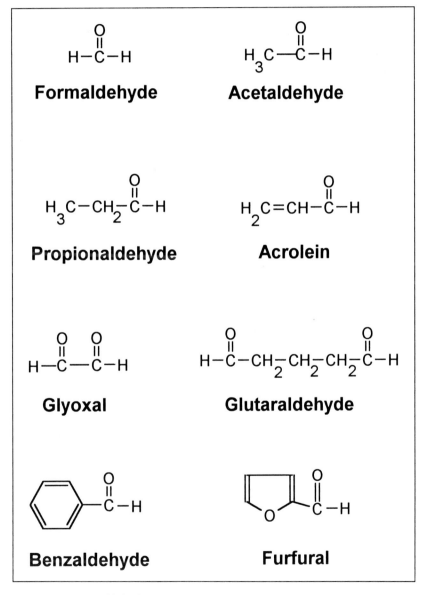

Fig. 5.1. Reactive aldehydes.

One model proposed for the formation of 40S intermediates by aphidicolin involves arrest of DNA polymerase movement while helicases and topoisomerases continue to unwind the parental DNA strands. This results in an extended, single stranded region at the replication fork. At some point, this single stranded region re-anneals, causing a replication intermediate with exceptionally high levels of negative superhelicity.[7] This model can account for the 40S intermediates caused by bifunctional aldehydes if it is assumed that DNA polymerase is stopped, either by being crosslinked directly to the DNA or by encountering chromosomal proteins crosslinked to the DNA. This variation of the model predicts that DNA helicase is not greatly affected by these aldehydes or by chromosomal proteins crosslinked to DNA. Although acrolein and formaldehyde can form adducts with DNA,[8,9] it is unlikely that these bifunctional aldehydes have any common adduct that could cause the 40S intermediate. The monofunctional aldehydes have the same reactive group and can form DNA adducts, yet do not cause 40S intermediates. This evidence strongly supports a causal effect between protein-DNA crosslinking and the formation of 40S intermediates.

Although 40S replication intermediates collapse and become inactivated, similar replication fork collapse in mammalian chromosomes might not inactivate a replicon. It is likely that the damaged DNA segment could still be replicated by a fork moving into it from an adjacent chromosomal replicon. However, the site of an arrested replication fork might not be replicated faithfully if accurate repair has not taken place.

Formaldehyde is known to cause DNA strand breaks[10] and was found to cause pronounced nicking of parental DNA strands in SV40 Cairns replication intermediates.[6] Replication forks were broken by collisions with these single strand breaks in a significant fraction of the viral replication intermediates. Similar double strand DNA breaks at replication forks are thought to be the basis for cytotoxicity and clastogenicity of the topoisomerase I poison camptothecin (chapter 3). Topoisomerase I is covalently linked to the DNA at the sites of camptothecin-induced DNA strand breaks. It is not known if the DNA strand breaks caused by formaldehyde are specifically associated with some of the protein crosslinked to the DNA.

Formaldehyde and acrolein caused accumulation of catenated SV40 daughter chromosomes, a signature of topoisomerase II inhibition (chapter 4). The inhibition of topoisomerase II by these bifunctional crosslinking agents could occur by several mechanisms. It is possible that topoisomerase II is sensitive to inactivation by formaldehyde. Formaldehyde is known to selectively inactivate the DNA repair enzyme O^6-methylguanine-DNA methyltransferase.[11] The inactivation could occur in several ways, such as reaction in the enzyme's active site or by crosslinking the two subunits and locking of the enzyme in an inactive conformation. Topoisomerase II activity may also depend on diffusion of the enzyme to new DNA "nodes" after each strand passing reaction. This diffusion could be limited by nonspecific formaldehyde crosslinking of the enzyme to DNA or by decreased one-dimensional diffusion of the enzyme on DNA due to histone-DNA crosslinks.

The specific disruptions of SV40 DNA replication caused by bifunctional aldehydes are consistent with the known mutagenicity and clastogenicity of these compounds. Arrest of SV40 DNA replication forks by the 40S pathway or by double strand breaks at the forks can initiate recombinational events which would cause rearrangements in cellular chromosomes.

ULTRAVIOLET (UV) RADIATION

For over a decade, the SV40 minichromosome has been used as a model to study the effects of UV damage on DNA replication. These studies were greatly facilitated by the availability of T4 UV endonuclease which cleaves DNA at cyclobutane pyrimidine dimers. Since these pyrimidine dimers are the major UV photolesion, it was assumed that other photolesions would be negligible at low UV fluences that produced only a few cyclobutane dimers per SV40 genome. Williams and Cleaver[12] observed that UV irradiation greatly decreased incorporation of thymidine label into replicating SV40 DNA. This was interpreted as inhibition of nascent DNA strand elongation by pyrimidine dimers. They noted that form I DNA synthesis was inhibited more than total SV40 DNA synthesis. During a 3 hr chase following UV doses estimated to give 1-2 pyrimidine dimers per SV40 genome, a significant amount of form I DNA was made. This was interpreted as meaning that replication forks can bypass pyrimidine dimers after initial blockage. Form II DNA did not accumulate. T4 UV endonuclease-sensitive sites in form I DNA decreased with time, suggesting that pyrimidine dimers in form I DNA might be repaired.[13] The efficiency of pyrimidine dimer formation was found to be the same in viral chromatin, previrions and virions.[14]

A temperature sensitive SV40 mutant was used to synchronize viral DNA replication in studies which found that replication was blocked on one side of the replication fork at the first pyrimidine dimer encountered, but that synthesis could continue on the other side of the replication fork.[15] A specific block to nascent strand synthesis on the leading strand side of the fork was suggested. Synthesis did not rapidly resume beyond the block, but there was eventual trans-dimer synthesis on the leading strand and gap filling on the lagging strand. Studies using aphidicolin to improve the synchronization of viral DNA in this system supported the idea that replication was blocked on the leading strand side (but not the lagging strand side) of a fork when a dimer was encountered on the leading strand.[16] In this model, dimers encountered on the lagging strand side cause only small gaps. Although some studies have found that Cairns replication intermediates are nicked after UV irradiation,[15,17] others have found that the parental DNA strands are intact.[18]

Stacks and coworkers found that the UV fluence-dependent decrease in SV40 DNA replication is largely due to a decrease in initiation of replication and a block in the progression of intermediates to form I.[19] They found that the percentage of completed molecules containing pyrimidine dimers increased with time until more than 50% contained dimers 3 hr after an irradiation of 40 J/m². An unusual approach taken by Barnett and coworkers involved mathematical model fitting, combined with a method for measuring the distribution of thymidine label in specific SV40 restriction fragments.[20] The results were interpreted as best fitting a model in which any pyrimidine dimer encountered by a replication fork prevents complete synthesis of the viral genome, and the block is independent of whether the dimer is on the leading or lagging strand side of the replication fork. White and Dixon reported that gap filling rather than replication fork progression is the rate limiting step in the replication of UV-damaged SV40 DNA.[21] This study also found no asymmetric pauses or blocks of replication forks. The replication forks in UV-irradiated Cairns replication intermediates were symmetrically located with respect to the origin of DNA replication. With or without UV-irradiation, Cairns replication intermediates disappeared at the same rate. Relaxed DNA circles (form II) were found to have randomly located gaps or nicks in the daughter DNA strands. Pulse-chase experiments showed that the fraction of SV40 replication intermediates passing through the nicked or gapped circular intermediate was a function of UV fluence.

Although electron microscopy studies by White and Dixon[21] found that replication forks are symmetric with respect to the replication origin following UV irradiation, a similar study by Berger and Edenberg found pronounced replication fork asymmetry.[22] Berger and Edenberg argued that a lesion on at least one side of the replication fork must block the replication forks, whereas a lesion on the other side would not. This interpretation favors models in which pyrimidine dimers on the leading strand side of the fork block its movement, while lagging strand dimers are bypassed, leaving a small gap.

Pre-irradiation of the host (monkey) cells was found to mitigate the effects of UV on SV40 DNA replication.[23] If cells were given a low UV exposure (5-10 J/m^2) before infection, a dose of 60 J/m^2 was required to inhibit SV40 DNA replication to the same extent as a dose of 25 J/m^2 in cells that were not irradiated before infection. The conclusion was that the effect was due, in part, to lowered UV inhibition of re-entry into DNA replication by replicated viral genomes in the pre-irradiated cells. Treger and coworkers also studied this phenomenon and concluded that it was not due to an expansion of the pool of replication intermediates.[24] They found that gapped form II DNA was the major product of SV40 DNA replication after UV fluences producing 1-3 pyrimidine dimers per SV40 genome. Pre-irradiation did not change the proportion of gapped form II molecules, so increased DNA synthesis past dimers without gaps was ruled out. The proportion of form I containing pyrimidine dimers was also unchanged by pre-irradiation. Pulse-chase experiments suggested that there was a more efficient conversion of gapped form II molecules to form I in the pre-irradiated cells. In subsequent studies of the pre-irradiation phenomenon, Scaria and Edenberg found that pre-irradiation of host cells did not alter blockage of SV40 DNA replication forks.[25] This finding was interpreted as ruling out removal of dimers, trans dimer DNA synthesis, or continued fork movement beyond dimers. Enhanced re-entry into DNA replication was suggested as the basis of the pre-irradiation effect.

Mezzina and coworkers reported evidence of growing fork blockage and single-stranded gaps in daughter strands after UV irradiation.[17] The blocked replication intermediates were found to be double strand DNA circles with double strand DNA tails (sigma forms). The double strand tail lengths were found to correspond to the inter-dimer distance as determined by T4 UV endonuclease. Normal Cairns replication intermediates (theta forms) were found in un-irradiated cells. Significant single strand gaps were seen in the replicated regions by several techniques. It was suggested that a repair endonuclease might be responsible for the DNA strand breaks. These results were interpreted in terms of blockage of DNA synthesis by lesions on the leading strand side of replication forks and trans-dimer synthesis (leaving a gap) for dimers on the lagging strand side. The effect of UV-irradiation has also been studied using in vitro SV40 DNA replication.[26] Although the unwinding of DNA by the SV40 large T antigen in vitro was not sensitive to UV damage, DNA synthesis was reduced to 35% of control levels by a UV dose producing 3-6 pyrimidine dimers per DNA circle. This study suggested that DNA synthesis proceeds past some lesions. Some of the problems of using an in vitro replication system for a study of this type were discussed.

Studies on the effects of UV on SV40 DNA replication have resulted in many contradictory reports, differing on a number of points. Very different conclusions and models have been drawn due to the methodology and protocols used. Low resolution techniques such as sucrose gradient centrifugation have been used extensively in these studies. Clearly, clean and indisputable results have been elusive. Most of these studies assume that pyrimidine dimers greatly exceed other UV photolesions. If this assumption were true, then pyrimidine dimers would be the only significant effectors of SV40 DNA replication at UV doses, causing only a few dimers per SV40 genome. However, the cytotoxic and mutagenic (6-4) photodimer may be present at half the levels of the pyrimidine dimers.[27] Also, it should be noted that most of the SV40 DNA replication intermediates at any one moment, for instance, during a short irradiation, are in the late stage of replication due to the well known slowing of replication fork movement as the terminus region is approached (chapter 4).

DNA ALKYLATING AGENTS

The SV40 DNA replication system has been used to understand how the carcinogen AAAF (*N*-acetoxyl-*N*-acetylaminofluorene) affects DNA replication in mammalian cells.[28] Viral DNA replication was severely inhibited, and Cairns replication intermediates were blocked from progressing to forms I and II. The nascent daughter strands, made after exposure to AAAF, had a length distribution equal to the average distance between AAAF-DNA adducts. Only 6% of the replication intermediates were normal theta-form Cairns structures after exposure to AAAF. The rest were mainly gapped DNA circles (72%) and DNA circles with double stranded DNA tails (sigma forms, 13%). Antibody to AAAF-guanine adducts was found to bind at the point where double strand DNA tails are attached to the circular part of the sigma form replication intermediates. The results were interpreted by a model in which replication forks were blocked by AAAF adducts on the leading strand sides, but not by adducts on the lagging strand sides.

The antileukemic xanthone psorospermin (Fig. 5.2) is isolated from the roots of *Psorospermum febrifugum*, a plant native to Africa.[29] This drug caused dose-dependent protein-DNA crosslinks to replicating SV40 DNA in vivo (Fig. 5.3). One dimensional agarose gel electrophoresis of the viral DNA replication intermediates from psorospermin-treated cells showed dose-dependent DNA nicking associated with a progressive decrease in electrophoretic mobility (Fig. 5.4, A, B). A similar nicking and electrophoretic shifting was seen when purified SV40 DNA was treated with psorospermin in vitro (Fig. 5.4, C). This shows that cellular proteins are not required for the DNA nicking or the decreased electrophoretic mobility of the viral DNA after exposure to psorospermin. The protein-DNA crosslinking in vivo must, therefore, be a secondary phenomenon. Psorospermin intercalates into DNA on the 5' side of guanine and alkylates the N7 position of guanine through the C4' carbon of its epoxide group.[30] At the time of the SV40 study, the DNA intercalation and alkylation were speculative. The progressive electrophoretic shifting was consistent with the addition of bulky alkylating groups to the DNA.

Analysis of psorospermin-treated SV40 DNA by two-dimensional neutral-alkaline gel electrophoresis (chapter 2) showed that form I DNA became nicked under the alkaline conditions of the second dimension gel electrophoresis. This indicated that the superhelical DNA harbored alkaline-sensitive sites after exposure to

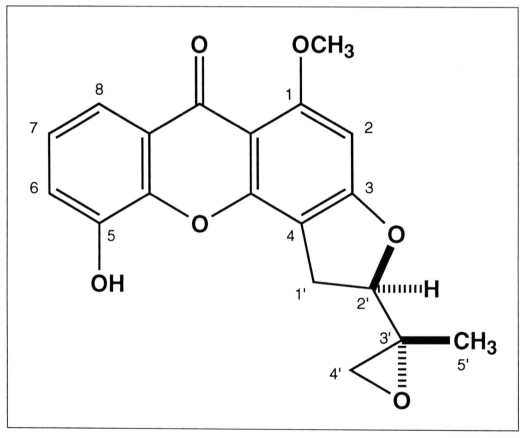

Fig. 5.2. Psorospermin. Reprinted from Cancer Res 1994; 54:3191, by permission of American Association for Cancer Research, Inc.

psorospermin. Alkylation of DNA bases is known to increase the rate of depurination,[31] and apurinic DNA sites are nicked in alkaline conditions. DNA can also lose pyrimidines, so abasic sites are sometimes called apurinic/apyrimidinic sites or A/P sites. Psorospermin-treated SV40 DNA was subjected to several specific tests for abasic sites. The amine groups of putrescine can react with abasic sites to form Schiff bases which can undergo β-elimination reactions to cause DNA strand breaks.[32] Heating with putrescine (45°C) in the presence of magnesium ion degraded SV40 DNA from psorospermin-treated cells to small genomic fragments,

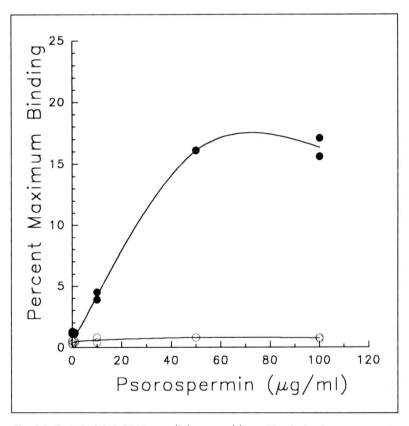

Fig. 5.3. Protein-SV40 DNA crosslinks caused by a 15 min in vivo exposure to psorospermin. The GF/C filter assay (chapter 2) for protein-DNA crosslinks was used to determine the fraction of pulse-labeled SV40 DNA crosslinked to protein. Hirt extract supernatants from the psorospermin-treated cells were assayed directly for protein-DNA crosslinks (●) or they were assayed after digestion with proteinase K (○). Reprinted from Cancer Res 1994; 54:3191, by permission of American Association for Cancer Research, Inc.

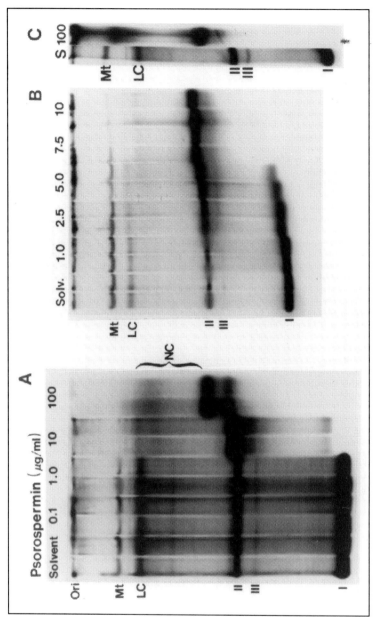

Fig. 5.4. Damage to SV40 DNA replication intermediates caused by psorospermin. Experiments were done in duplicate and placed in adjacent lanes for one-dimensional agarose gel electrophoresis. The psorospermin concentration used is indicated above each pair of duplicate lanes. SV40-infected CV-1 cells were labeled with tritiated thymidine (30 min, 250 μCi/ml) at 36 hr post-infection. The drug or its solvent was added 15 min after the start of labeling. The viral DNA replication intermediates were then extracted and prepared for electrophoresis (chapter 2). A, Dose-response for 15 min exposures to psorospermin. B, Same, but covering the concentration range 1.0-10 μg/ml. C, treatment of purified SV40 DNA for 1 hr with psorospermin (100 μg/ml). Abbreviations: Ori, origin of electrophoresis; Mt, mitochondrial DNA; LC, late Cairns structures; II, form II (nicked circle) DNA; III, form III (double strand linear) DNA; I, form I (superhelical circle) DNA; NC, nicked Cairns structures. Normal intermediate Cairns structures make up the continuous smear extending from the form I band to the LC band (chapter 2). Reprinted from Cancer Res 1994, 54:3191, by permission of American Association for Cancer Research, Inc.

but had no effect on DNA from untreated cells. Endonuclease IV, an abasic site-specific endonuclease, also reduced viral DNA from psorospermin-treated cells to subgenomic fragments without affecting the DNA from untreated cells (Fig. 5.5). These results show that psorospermin causes extensive depurination of SV40 DNA replication intermediates in vivo.

Although it is possible that psorospermin nicks DNA directly, DNA strand breaks can occur at abasic sites by reactions with amine groups in proteins and other molecules. The nicking occurs by Schiff base formation and β-elimination as in the putrescine reaction. The Schiff base is a covalent intermediate which can be made irreversible by reduction. One strategy for footprinting chromosomal proteins involves DNA alkylation with dimethyl sulfate and heating to cause loss of the alkylated bases. The resulting abasic sites react with amine groups of chromosomal proteins to form protein-DNA crosslinks.[33] Calf thymus topoisomerase I and topoisomerase II formed crosslinks to purified SV40 DNA in vitro, as did purified *Drosophila* topoisomerase II.[34] However, cytochrome C also formed crosslinks to psorospermin-treated DNA, suggesting a nonspecific mechanism of DNA crosslinking to DNA-binding proteins. While these data do not rule out the possibility that psorospermin or psorospermin-induced abasic sites may stabilize topoisomerase-DNA cleavable complexes, the crosslinking of cytochrome C suggests that nonspecific mechanisms must at least contribute to the in vivo protein-DNA crosslinking of psorospermin.

Adozelesin (Fig. 5.6) is a synthetic analog of CC-1065, an extremely cytotoxic antibiotic isolated from the fermentation broth of *Streptomyces zelensis*.[35] CC-1065 had significant antineoplastic activity but caused delayed cell death.[36] Adozelesin shows good activity against a wide variety of tumors, but does not cause delayed cell death like its parent compound.[37] CC-1065 is a minor groove DNA binding agent with a specificity for AT-rich regions. It alkylates mainly the N-3 position of adenine, and the adenine-CC-1065 adduct can be released by heating at 90-100°C.[38] DNA strand breakage occurs spontaneously at the resulting abasic sites.[39,40]

SV40 DNA extracted from cells treated with adozelesin showed a dose-dependent DNA nicking (Fig. 5.7). At the lowest dose tested

Fig. 5.5. Endonuclease IV digestion of SV40 DNA replication intermediates from untreated control cells or from cells treated with psorospermin. Experiments were done in duplicate. ⊕, digestion with endonuclease IV; ⊖, mock digestion (no endonuclease). Reaction mixtures (50 µl) contained 20 µg/ml of SV40 DNA from cells treated with the solvent dimethyl sulfoxide alone (Control) or with psorospermin (50 µg/ml, 15 min). Reprinted from Cancer Res 1994; 54:3191, by permission of American Association for Cancer Research, Inc.

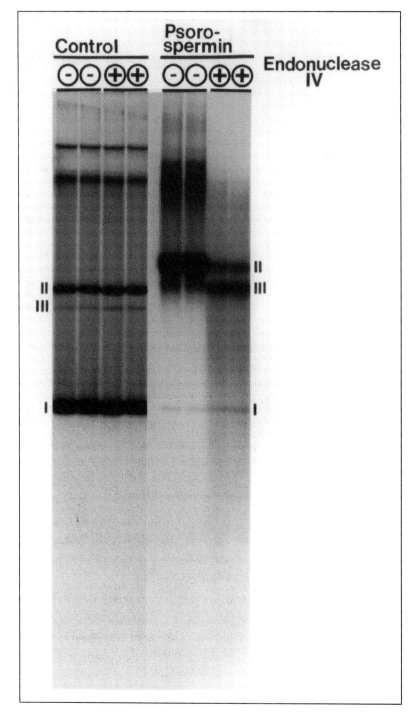

(0.5 μg/ml), there was a marked decrease in label in the late Cairns structure and an increase in label in the form II band and in the region between the form I and III bands. Adozelesin treatment also caused low-level SV40 DNA-protein crosslinks as measured by the GF/C filter binding assay (Fig. 5.8). The DNA nicking and protein-DNA crosslinking were reminiscent of the psorospermin results except that there was no dose-dependent decrease in the electrophoretic mobility of the viral replication intermediates. The accumulation of label in the region between the form I and III bands is suggestive of 40S intermediates (chapter 3). However, there was not a clear and well-defined 40S band.

Two-dimensional neutral-alkaline gel electrophoresis of SV40 DNA replication intermediates from adozelesin-treated cells showed pronounced vertical streaks from the completely replicated forms I, II and III (Fig. 5.9). Small vertical streaks are often associated with forms II and III in the alkaline second dimension. They are due to pre-existing single strand breaks which are only revealed under denaturing conditions. A DNA strand break converts form I to form II, however, form II may have many single strand breaks in either the daughter or parental DNA strands. In the same way,

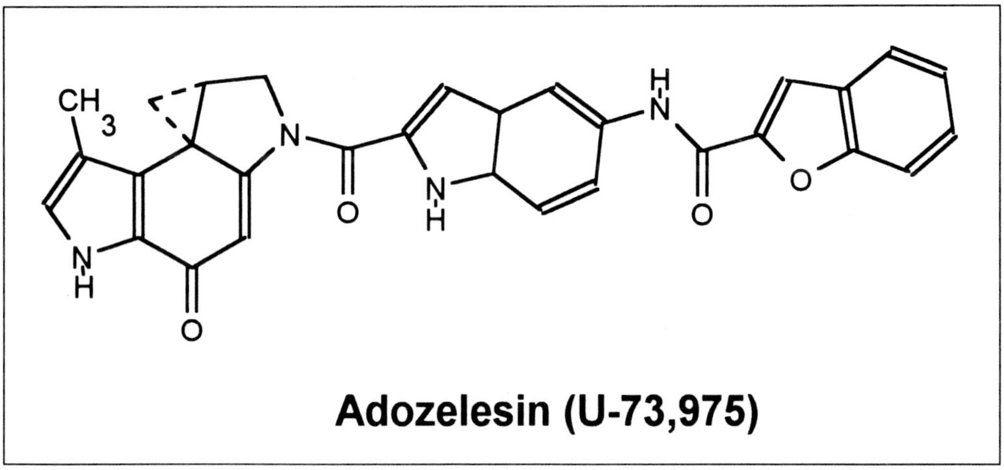

Adozelesin (U-73,975)

Fig. 5.6. Adozelesin (also known as U-73975). Adozelesin was a kind gift of J. Patrick McGovren, Upjohn Laboratories.

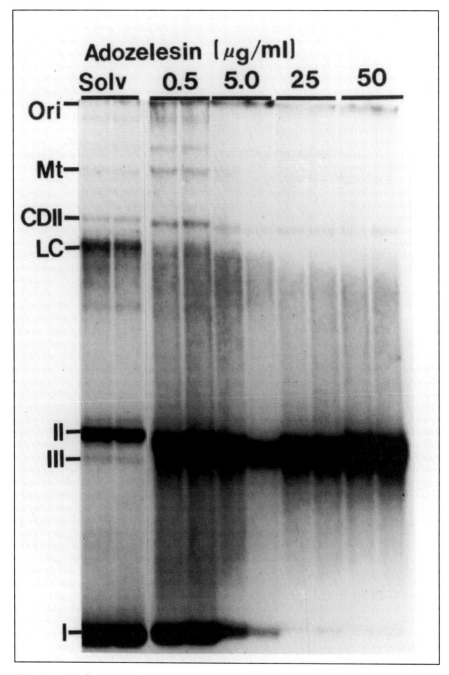

Fig. 5.7. One-dimensional agarose gel electrophoresis of pulse-labeled SV40 DNA extracted from cells exposed to adozelesin. Abbreviations: Solv., solvent (dimethyl sulfoxide) control for the highest concentration of adozelesin used; CDII, form II circular (head-to-tail) dimer (see chapter 8). Other abbreviations are the same as in Figure 5.4.

the electrophoretic mobility of form III DNA under neutral conditions is not affected by the presence of numerous additional single strand breaks. As seen in the untreated control (Fig. 5.9, top), the vertical streaks are not normally associated with form I DNA. By definition, form I DNA cannot have hidden single strand breaks. However, the form I band from the adozelesin-treated cells showed a pronounced vertical streak in the alkaline second dimension (Fig. 5.9, middle). This means that the form I SV40 DNA from adozelesin-treated cells did have DNA strand breaks under the

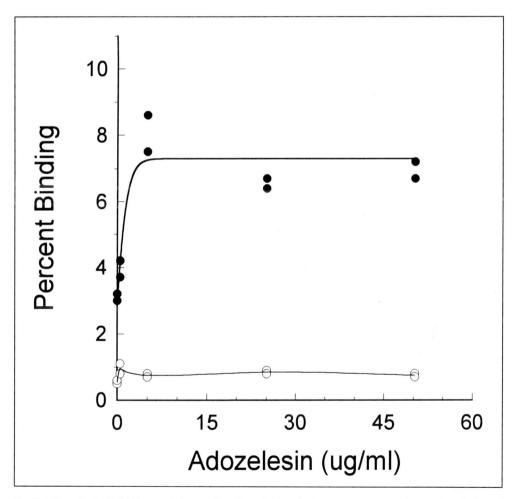

Fig. 5.8. Protein-SV40 DNA crosslinks as a function of adozelesin concentration in the media of infected cells (15 min exposure).

Fig. 5.9. Two-dimensional neutral-alkaline gel electrophoresis of SV40 DNA replication intermediates from adozelesin-treated cells and untreated control cells. The first dimension separation is identical to that shown in Figure 5.7, and a duplicate first dimension lane (run left to right) is shown across the top of the corresponding alkaline second dimension separation (run top to bottom). Abbreviations: IC, intermediate Cairns structures; B1, B-family catenated SV40 daughter chromosomes; C, unresolved C-family catenated SV40 daughter chromosomes and form I circular (head-to-tail) dimers; 40S, torsionally stressed replication intermediates. Other abbreviations are the same as in Figures 5.4, 5.7 and 5.9. 40S intermediates are discussed in chapter 3, catenated dimers in chapter 4, and circular dimers in chapter 8.

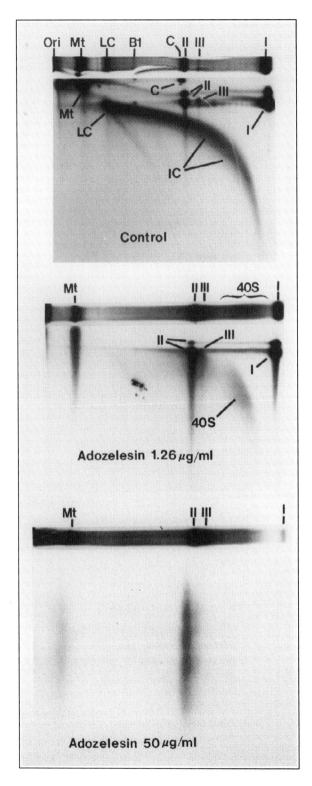

alkaline conditions of the second dimension gel. As with psoro-spermin, this is suggestive of abasic sites. Forms II and III from the adozelesin-treated cells were also extensively degraded in alkaline buffer. Normal Cairns replication intermediates were not evident in the adozelesin-treated samples, but there was a remnant of 40S replication intermediates. Higher doses of adozelesin caused very extensive nicking of SV40 intermediates, and the nicked intermediates contained large numbers of alkaline-sensitive sites as shown by extensive degradation in alkaline conditions (Fig. 5.9, bottom).

Two-dimensional neutral-chloroquine gel analysis of SV40 DNA from adozelesin-treated cells confirmed the formation of 40S intermediates (Fig. 5.10). After an adozelesin exposure of 1.26 µg/ml, the growing replication intermediates were present in four forms. A remnant of normal intermediate Cairns structures (IC) could be seen as an arc extending from the late Cairns structure to the form I band (Fig. 5.10, middle). An arc of nicked Cairns structures extended from the late Cairns band to the form II DNA band. Sigma forms with a single broken replication fork also extended back from the form II band (LC). The remainder of the replication intermediates were present as 40S structures and forms intermediate between 40S and normal intermediate Cairns structures. These forms were largely lost due to degradation in the alkaline second dimension gel as shown in Figure 5.9.

Although abasic sites in DNA are alkali labile, alkali lability alone is not proof of abasic sites. To confirm the presence of abasic sites, SV40 DNA replication intermediates from untreated control cells and from adozelesin-exposed cells were treated with purified endonuclease IV (Fig. 5.11). Endonuclease IV cleaves DNA specifically at abasic sites.[41-43] The viral DNA from adozelesin-treated cells was partially degraded by endonuclease IV, indicating that many of the alkali sensitive sites are abasic sites. Periodicity in the subgenomic degradation products resembled a nucleosomal DNA ladder and suggests that chromatin structure may influence either alkylation of DNA by adozelesin or loss of the modified bases. Abasic sites, DNA strand breaks and protein-DNA crosslinks are all well known cytotoxic DNA lesions. Although these lesions are likely to contribute to the cytotoxicity of adozelesin, other

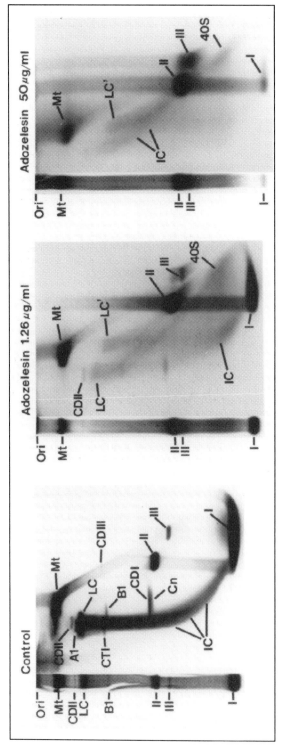

Fig. 5.10. Two-dimensional neutral-chloroquine gel electrophoresis of SV40 DNA replication intermediates from adozelesin-treated cells. The first dimension separations were done as in Figure 5.7, and are shown (run top to bottom) to the left of the corresponding chloroquine second dimension (shown run left to right). Abbreviations: CDI, form I circular dimer; CDII, form III (linearized) circular dimer; A1, A-family catenated SV40 daughter chromosomes; CTI, form I circular trimer; LC', sigma-form replication intermediates with one broken replication fork; Cn, C-family catenated SV40 daughter chromosomes with catenation linking numbers one and above (partially resolved from the form I circular dimer band). Other abbreviations are the same as in Figures 5.4, 5.7 and 5.9.

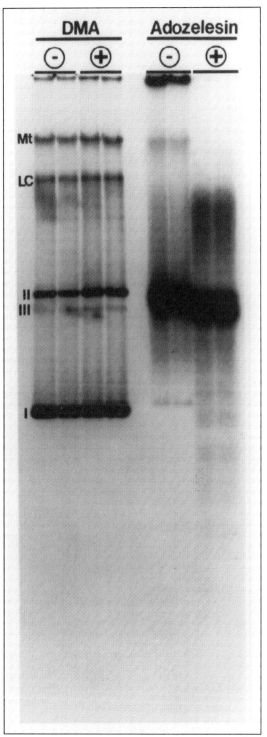

Fig. 5.11. Endonuclease IV digestion of SV40 DNA replication intermediates from untreated control cells or from cells treated with adozelesin. Experiments were done in duplicate. ⊕, digestion with endonuclease IV; ⊖, mock digestion (no endonuclease). Infected cells were treated with 50 μg/ml adozelesin, 30 min, 37 °C.

adozelesin-induced DNA lesions may make greater contributions to the cytotoxicity or anticancer activity of adozelesin. SV40 DNA from adozelesin-treated cells had many alkali-labile sites, but endonuclease IV caused only a partial digestion of the modified DNA, suggesting that some alkali-labile sites may not be abasic sites. The protein-DNA crosslinking caused by adozelesin was low compared to that caused by psorospermin.

Some of the effects of psorospermin and adozelesin on SV40 DNA replication may be due to the DNA binding properties of these drugs or to their bulk as DNA adducts. To understand how small, simple alkylating agents affect SV40 DNA replication, infected cells were treated with dimethyl sulfate (Fig. 5.12). Very high concentrations of dimethyl sulfate were required to disrupt SV40 DNA replication in the standard assay. At high concentrations of dimethyl sulfate (1.0-10 mM), 40S intermediates were produced. At higher concentrations there was extensive nicking of replication intermediates. No protein-DNA crosslinks were detected at any concentration of dimethyl sulfate. This is probably because heating is required for extensive depurination of dimethyl sulfate modified DNA. The DNA was heated at 45°C during deproteinization before gel electrophoresis. This heating was similar to the heating step used by Levina and coworkers to depurinate dimethyl sulfate-treated chromatin.[33]

Although the SV40 DNA replication system has many advantages for studies of DNA damaging agents, the studies tend to be complicated by several factors. DNA damage by both physical and chemical agents tends to be heterogeneous. The assumption that the effects on SV40 DNA replication are due to the major lesion is questionable. Minor lesions may disrupt DNA replication more efficiently than major lesions. To understand the effect of a specific lesion, special reagents such as DNA damage-specific antibodies or damage-specific endonucleases are used. Even the use of these tools may be complicated by modifications of DNA structure such as single strand gaps. It is important to know if the endonuclease or antibody recognizes the DNA lesion in both single stranded and double stranded DNA. DNA lesions may also have very different effects depending on their location on the leading or lagging strand sides of replication forks. Since damage from chemical and physical agents goes into the DNA randomly, this problem might be approached using an in vitro SV40 DNA replication system which makes use of an artificial template modified to contain specific types of damage in specific locations.

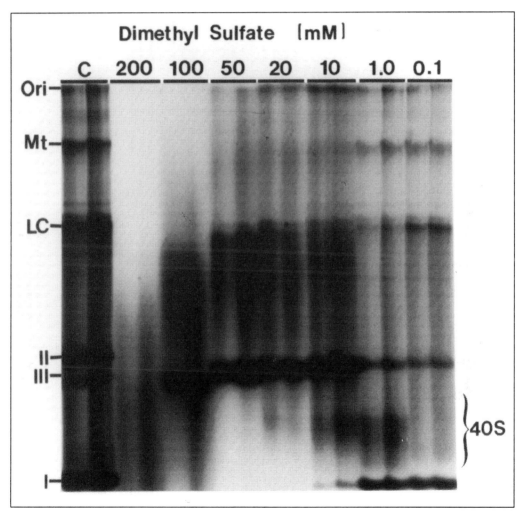

Fig. 5.12. One dimensional agarose gel electrophoresis of SV40 DNA replication intermediates resulting from exposure to dimethyl sulfate. SV40-infected cells were exposed to the indicated concentrations of dimethyl sulfate for the last 15 min of a 30 min labeling with tritiated thymidine. The SV40 DNA in the Hirt extract supernatant was deproteinized by digestion with proteinase K (4 hr at 45°C) and chloroform isopropanol extraction before electrophoresis.

REFERENCES

1. Snapka RM. Topoisomerase inhibitors can selectively interfere with different stages of simian virus 40 DNA replication. Mol Cell Biol 1986; 6:4221-4227.
2. Ma T-H, Harris MM. Review of the genotoxicity of formaldehyde. Mutat Res 1988; 196:37-59.
3. Nelson N, Levine RJ, Albert RE et al. Contribution of formaldehyde to respiratory cancer. Env Health Perspect 1986; 70:23-35.
4. Kuykendall JR, Bogdanffy MS. Efficiency of DNA-histone crosslinking induced by saturated and unsaturated aldehydes in vitro. Mut Res 1992; 283:131-136.
5. Feron VJ, Til HP, de Vrijer F et al. Aldehydes: occurrence, carcinogenic potential, mechanism of action and risk assessment. Mutat Res 1991; 259:363-385.
6. Permana PA, Snapka RM. Aldehyde-induced protein-DNA crosslinks disrupt specific stages of SV40 DNA replication. Carcinogenesis 1994; 15:1031-1036.
7. Dröge P, Sogo JM, Stahl H. Inhibition of DNA synthesis by aphidicolin induces supercoiling in simian virus 40 replicative intermediates. EMBO J 1985; 4:3241-3246.
8. Randerath K, Reddy MV, Gupta RC. ^{32}P-labeling test for DNA damage. Proc Natl Acad Sci USA 1981; 78:6126-6129.
9. Povey AC, Cooper DP, Littler E. ^{32}P-Postlabeling of alkylated thymidines using Epstein-Barr virus encoded thymidine kinase. Carcinogenesis 1991; 12:709-712.
10. Auerbach C, Moutschen-Dahmen M, Moutschen J. Genetic and cytogenetic effects of formaldehyde and related compounds. Mutat Res 1977; 39:317-362.
11. Krokan H, Grafstrom RC, Sundqvist K et al. Cytotoxicity, thiol depletion and inhibition of O^6-methylguanine-DNA methyltransferase by various aldehydes in cultured human bronchial fibroblasts. Carcinogenesis 1985; 6:1755-1759.
12. Williams JI, Cleaver JE. Perturbations in simian virus 40 DNA synthesis by ultraviolet light. Mutat Res 1978; 52:301-311.
13. Williams JI, Cleaver JE. Removal of T4 endonuclease V-sensitive sites from SV40 DNA after exposure to ultraviolet light. Biochim Biophys Acta 1979; 562:429-437.
14. Edenberg HJ, Roman A. Introduction of pyrimidine dimers into different intracellular forms of simian virus 40. Photochem Photobiol 1983; 37:297-299.
15. Sarasin AR, Hanawalt PC. Replication of ultraviolet-irradiated simian virus 40 in monkey kidney cells. J Mol Biol 1980; 138:299-319.
16. Clark JM, Hanawalt PC. Replicative intermediates in UV-irradiated simian virus 40. Mutat Res 1984; 132:1-14.

17. Mezzina M, Menck CFM, Courtin P et al. Replication of simian virus 40 DNA after UV irradiation: evidence of growing fork blockage and single-stranded gaps in daughter strands. J Virol 1988; 62:4249-4258.
18. Edenberg HJ. Inhibition of simian virus 40 DNA replication by ultraviolet light. Virology 1983; 128:298-309.
19. Stacks PC, White JH, Dixon K. Accommodation of pyrimidine dimers during replication of UV-damaged simian virus 40 DNA. Mol Cell Biol 1983; 3:1403-1411.
20. Barnett SW, Landaw EM, Dixon K. Test of models for replication of simian virus 40 DNA following ultraviolet irradiation. Biophys J 1984; 46:307-321.
21. White JH, Dixon K. Gap filling and not replication fork progression is the rate limiting step in the replication of UV-damaged simian virus 40 DNA. Mol Cell Biol 1984; 4:1286-1292.
22. Berger CA, Edenberg HJ. Pyrimidine dimers block simian virus 40 replication forks. Mol Cell Biol 1986; 6:3443-3450.
23. Scaria A, Edenberg HJ. Preirradiation of host (monkey) cells mitigates the effects of UV upon simian virus 40 DNA replication. Mutat Res 1987; 183:265-271.
24. Treger JM, Hauser J, Dixon K. Molecular analysis of enhanced replication of UV-damaged simian virus 40 DNA in UV-treated mammalian cells. Mol Cell Biol 1988; 8:2428-2434.
25. Scaria A, Edenberg HJ. Preirradiation of host cells does not alter blockage of simian virus 40 replication by pyrimidine dimers. Mutat Res 1988; 193:11-20.
26. Gough G, Wood RD. Inhibition of in vitro SV40 DNA replication by ultraviolet light. Mutat Res 1989; 227:193-197.
27. Mitchell DL, Allison JP, Nair RS. Immunoprecipitation of pyrimidine (6- 4)pyrimidone photoproducts and cyclobutane pyrimidine dimers in UV-irradiated DNA. Radiat Res 1990; 123:299-303.
28. Armier J, Mezzina M, Fuchs RPP et al. N-Acetoxy-N-2-acetylaminofluorene-induced damage on SV40 DNA: inhibition of DNA replication and visualization of DNA lesions. Carcinogenesis 1988; 9:789-795.
29. Kupchan SM, Streelman DR, Sneden A. Psorospermin, a new antileukemic xanthone from *Psorospermun febrifugum*. J Natural Prod 1980; 43:296-301.
30. Hansen M, Lee S-J, Cassady JM, Hurley C. Psorospermin intercalates into the DNA helix to position an epoxide into the major groove for electrophilic attack on N7 of guanine. Submitted.
31. Loeb L, Preston BD. Mutagenesis by apurinic/apyrimidinic sites. Ann Rev Genet 1986; 20:201-230.

32. Lindahl T, Andersson A. Rate of chain breakage at apurinic sites in double-stranded deoxyribonucleic acid. Biochemistry 1972; 11:3618-3622.

33. Levina ES, Bavykin SG, Shick VV et al. The method of crosslinking histones to DNA partly depurinated at neutral pH. Anal Biochem 1981; 110:93-101.

34. Permana PA, Ho DK, Cassady JM et al. Mechanism of action of the antileukemic xanthone psorospermin: DNA strand breaks, abasic sites and protein-DNA crosslinks. Cancer Res 1994; 54:3191-3195.

35. Bhuyan BK, Smith KS, Kelly RC et al. Multidrug resistance is a component of V79 cell resistance to the alkylating agent adozelesin. Cancer Res 1993; 53:1354-1359.

36. Warpehoski MA. Dissecting the complex structure of CC-1065. Drugs of the Future 1991; 16:131-141.

37. Li LH, Kelly RC, Warpehoski MA et al. Adozelesin, a selected lead among cyclopropylpyrroloindole analogs of the DNA-binding antibiotic, CC-1065. Invest New Drugs 1991; 9:137-148.

38. Hurley LH, Reynolds VL, Swenson DH et al. Reaction of the antitumor antibiotic CC-1065 with DNA: structure of a DNA adduct with DNA sequence specificity. Science 1984; 226:843-844.

39. Reynolds VL, Molineux IJ, Kaplan DJ et al. Reaction of the antitumor antibiotic CC-1065 with DNA. Location of the site of thermally induced breakage and analysis of DNA specificity. Biochemistry 1985; 24:6228-6237.

40. Zsido TJ, Woynarowski JM, Baker RM et al. Induction of heat-labile sites in DNA of mammalian cells by the antitumor alkylating agent CC-1065. Biochemistry 1991; 30:3733-3738.

41. Ljungquist S. A new endonuclease from *Escherichia coli* acting at apurinic sites in DNA. J Biol Chem 1977; 252:2808-2814.

42. Levin JD, Johnson AW, Demple B. Homogeneous *Escherichia coli* endonuclease IV. J Biol Chem 1988; 263:8066-8071.

43. Levin JD, Shapiro R, Demple B. Metalloenzymes in DNA repair. *Escherichia coli* endonuclease IV and *Saccharomyces cerevisiae* Apn1. J Biol Chem 1991; 266:22893-22898.

=========== CHAPTER 6 ===========

DRUG DISCOVERY
AND EVALUATION WITH SV40

Robert M. Snapka, Christopher A. Ferrer, Nan-Jun Sun
and John M. Cassady

SV40 in vivo DNA replication can be used as a powerful and informative assay for the discovery of drugs which disrupt DNA replication in mammalian cells. Many anticancer drugs are in this class—rapidly entering cells and disrupting DNA replication. The SV40 assay system can detect anticancer drugs in crude extracts of bioactive plants and at the same time provide mechanistic information which is used to prioritize the plants for continued fractionation and purification of active components. Purified enzymes and substrates are not required. The SV40 assay system is also insensitive to many natural products which cause false positives in cytotoxicity assays and assays involving purified enzymes.

Drugs which interfere with mammalian DNA replication cause distinctive "signature patterns" of aberrant SV40 DNA replication intermediates (Fig. 6.1). These patterns indicate the intracellular target and mechanism of the drug being tested: topoisomerase I poison, topoisomerase II poison, topoisomerase II antagonist, DNA polymerase inhibitor, DNA nicking agent, protein-DNA crosslinker, protein synthesis inhibitor or DNA alkylating agent. Known agents which give these signature patterns of aberrant SV40 replication intermediates are camptothecin, 4'-[9-acridinylamino]methane-sulfon-*m*-aniside (m-AMSA), ICRF-193, aphidicolin, bleomycin,

The SV40 Replicon Model for Analysis of Anticancer Drugs,
edited by Robert M. Snapka. ©1996 R.G. Landes Company.

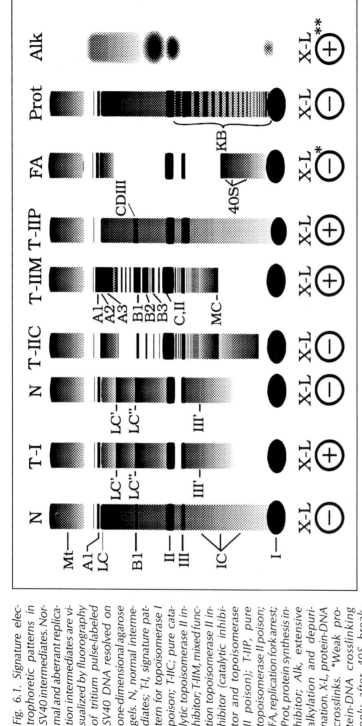

Fig. 6.1. Signature electrophoretic patterns in SV40 intermediates. Normal and aberrant replication intermediates are visualized by fluorography of tritium pulse-labeled SV40 DNA resolved on one-dimensional agarose gels. N, normal intermediates; T-I, signature pattern for topoisomerase I poison; T-IIC, pure catalytic topoisomerase II inhibitor; T-IIM, mixed function topoisomerase II inhibitor (catalytic inhibitor and topoisomerase II poison); T-IIP, pure topoisomerase II poison; FA, replication fork arrest; Prot, protein synthesis inhibitor; Alk, extensive alkylation and depurination. X-L, protein-DNA crosslinks. *Weak protein-DNA crosslinking only after 40S breakdown; **Protein-DNA crosslinking with strong depurination in vivo. I, form I (superhelical) DNA; II, form II (nicked circular) DNA; III, form III (linear) DNA; IC, intermediate Cairns structures (superhelical replication intermediates); LC, late Cairns structure (95% completed "figure 8" replication form); LC' & LC'', replication intermediates with one or two broken DNA replication forks respectively; III', linear forms resulting from two broken replication forks; 40S, torsionally stressed DNA replication intermediates; A1-A3, nicked-nicked catenated daughter chromosomes with catenation linking number indicated; B1-B3, nicked-superhelical catenated daughter chromosomes with catenation linking number indicated; CDIII, circular dimer form III (linear); MC, unresolved B-family dimers; KB, Keller bands (form I with low supercoiling); C, C-family (superhelical-superhelical) catenated dimers (unresolved).

formaldehyde, cycloheximide and dimethyl sulfate, respectively. In order to disrupt SV40 DNA replication and produce a signature pattern, drugs must cross the cell membrane and reach the nucleus within a few minutes. Agents which do not readily cross membranes do not affect SV40 in vivo DNA replication in this assay. This means that the SV40 replication system is unaffected by most tannins, complex alcohols, charged polymers and other natural products which can interfere with both cytotoxicity-based screens and mechanism-based assays using purified enzymes or receptors. The SV40 assay system is also insensitive to drugs which target microtubules, mitochondria, membranes and other cellular targets. In this sense, SV40 in vivo replication is intermediate between cytotoxicity-based screens and narrowly focused mechanism-based screens for the discovery of anticancer drugs. The SV40 DNA replication assay might be described as a mechanism-group-based screen for agents disrupting DNA replication in mammalian cells.

TOPOISOMERASE I POISON SIGNATURE PATTERN

The most prominent features of the topoisomerase I poison signature pattern are due to DNA replication fork breaks.[1,2] When moving replication forks encounter drug-stabilized topoisomerase I-DNA cleavage complexes, a double strand break occurs (see earlier discussion in chapter 3). As a result, the smear of normal replication intermediates is replaced by three shorter smears of intermediates resulting from either one replication fork break (LC') or two replication fork breaks (LC" and III', Fig. 6.1). Since these intermediates are all crosslinked to protein (the covalent topoisomerase I-DNA linkage),[3] the tritium pulsed-labeled SV40 DNA is retained on GF/C filters in 0.4 M guanidinium chloride.[4] The topoisomerase I poison signature pattern consists of the replacement of normal replication intermediates by forms with broken replication forks and a high level of protein crosslinking to the pulse-labeled viral genomes.

TOPOISOMERASE II INHIBITION AND POISONING

Inhibition of topoisomerase II slows the topoisomerase II-dependent steps of SV40 DNA replication — replication of the terminus region and decatenation of the daughter chromosomes (see chapter 4 for detailed discussion). Topoisomerase poisoning is due to inhibition of the specific steps involved in DNA strand passing, often the religation step. However, inhibition can occur at other steps in the topoisomerase reaction such as DNA binding, consensus site recognition, or even by drug binding to the topoisomerase itself. "Pre-DNA cleavage" inhibitors or "catalytic inhibitors" can efficiently slow both the replication of the terminus region and decatenation. This type of inhibitor can also reduce DNA cleavage by topoisomerase II below the background level[5] and can reduce the enhancement of topoisomerase II-dependent DNA cleavage caused by topoisomerase II poisons.[4,5] In this sense, these drugs may be considered topoisomerase II antagonists.[4]

These two aspects of topoisomerase II inhibition, catalytic inhibition and topoisomerase poisoning, tend to vary inversely in the SV40 DNA replication system. The strongest in vivo catalytic inhibitors of topoisomerase II, as estimated by inhibition of topoisomerase II-dependent steps of SV40 DNA replication, tend to be the weakest topoisomerase II poisons. This is apparently because the strongest catalytic inhibitors of topoisomerase II tend to inhibit pre-DNA cleavage steps of the topoisomerase II reaction. Pure topoisomerase II antagonists or catalytic inhibitors cause accumulation of catenated SV40 dimers without stabilizing the "cleavable complex" DNA strand passing intermediate. Since there is no stabilization of the cleavable complex, there are no topoisomerase II-dependent DNA strand breaks or protein-DNA crosslinks. This pattern is diagrammed as "T-IIC" in Figure 6.1. Drugs in this class, including ICRF-193 analogs[6] and quinobenoxazines,[7] have shown anticancer activity. An additional diagnostic test for such drugs is that they prevent strong topoisomerase II poisons such as VP-16 from stabilizing topoisomerase II-DNA cleavage complexes.

Some of the strong topoisomerase II poisons, such as the quinolones CP-115,953 and CP-67,804,[8] cause no accumulation of catenated SV40 dimers or late Cairns replication intermediates—the in vivo indicators of topoisomerase II catalytic inhibition. This subgroup of strong topoisomerase II poisons causes only double strand DNA breaks in SV40 chromosomes to produce a greatly increased form III band relative to untreated controls. Since these are topoisomerase poisons, there is a strong dose-dependent protein-DNA crosslinking signal (Fig. 6.1). This "pure topoisomerase II poison" pattern is shown as "T-IIP" in Figure 6.1. The designation "pure topoisomerase II poison" does not mean that these drugs do not inhibit catalysis by topoisomerase II, but that the indications of catalytic inhibition are not evident in SV40 DNA replication intermediates. These drugs do cause inhibition of in vitro topoisomerase II reactions with purified enzymes and DNA substrates. In these in vitro reactions, topoisomerase II may be present in excess so that the DNA strand passing step of the topoisomerase II reaction, rather than pre-DNA cleavage steps, is rate limiting. The reverse may be true in vivo.

Most topoisomerase II inhibitors are "mixed function" inhibitors that inhibit intracellular topoisomerase II reactions and stabilize "cleavable complexes." The cleavable complexes stabilized in SV40 DNA in vivo by drugs like Adriamycin, m-AMSA and VM-26 have single strand DNA breaks rather than double strand breaks. Topoisomerase poisoning is indicated by high levels of protein-SV40 DNA crosslinking, and topoisomerase II inhibition is indicated by the accumulation of highly catenated SV40 daughter chromosomes and late Cairns structures (T-IIM in Fig. 6.1). Increasing concentrations of the drug cause progressively higher levels of protein-DNA crosslinking and catenated dimers with progressively higher catenation linking numbers. At high concentrations, the DNA-binding drugs can inhibit their own topoisomerase II poisoning (self-inhibition). The fact that topoisomerase II inhibitors can have anticancer activity without stabilizing cleavable complexes strongly suggests that inhibition of topoisomerase II-dependent steps in DNA replication contribute to the antineoplastic activity of these compounds. The relative contributions of topoisomerase II poisoning and topoisomerase II catalytic inhibition to nonspecific cytotoxicity and to selective activity against cancer cells remain largely unexplored for mixed function topoisomerase II inhibitors.

INHIBITION OF PROTEIN SYNTHESIS

Inhibitors of protein synthesis block the synthesis of new histones during DNA replication, resulting in loss of nucleosome structure in newly replicated SV40 daughter chromosomes. Since superhelicity in form I SV40 DNA is due to nucleosome structure, one negative superhelical turn per nucleosome (discussed in chapter 1), this loss of nucleosome structure results in form I DNA with lower than normal levels of supercoiling. Covalently closed SV40 DNAs with one to about 14 superhelical turns are distributed in a series of distinct bands between the position of the form I DNA band and the form II DNA band in one dimensional gel patterns. These "Keller" bands are diagnostic of disrupted nucleosome structure due to inhibition of protein synthesis (Prot, Fig. 6.1).

DNA REPLICATION FORK ARREST

Inhibition of DNA polymerases involved in SV40 replication causes the rapid formation of torsionally stressed 40S DNA replication intermediates.[9,10] Normal replication intermediates rapidly become "super-superhelical" and migrate collectively in a broad band just behind the form I band in one dimensional agarose gel electrophoretic patterns. These 40S intermediates spontaneously break down in vivo with the formation of DNA strand breaks and protein-DNA crosslinks (chapter 3). The breakdown begins as the intermediates form, so the appearance of a 40S band in the electrophoretic pattern is usually accompanied by detectable (but low level) protein-DNA crosslinking. The protein-DNA crosslinking reaches its maximum as breakdown of the 40S intermediates is completed. The maximum protein-DNA crosslinking in this case is about 8-9%, which is still low compared to the crosslinking caused by strong topoisomerase poisons or by direct protein-DNA crosslinking agents. The DNA nicking associated with breakdown of the 40S intermediates converts them to nicked Cairns replication intermediates which migrate between the position of the late Cairns structure and the form II DNA band in one dimensional gel patterns (chapter 2). The 40S structure forms rapidly but breaks down slowly, so it is seen whenever DNA polymerases are inhibited. A very prolonged exposure, on the order of an hour, to a DNA polymerase inhibitor would show only nicked Cairns structures and a high protein-DNA crosslink signal due to complete 40S breakdown. Since protein-DNA crosslinks (see below and chapter 5) and bulky alkylating agents (see adozelesin, chapter 5) can also cause 40S intermediates, they are probably a sign of DNA replication fork arrest rather than a sign of specific DNA polymerase inhibition (FA, Fig. 6.1).

PROTEIN-DNA CROSSLINKERS

As expected, direct protein-DNA crosslinking agents such as formaldehyde give very high protein-DNA crosslinking signals in the SV40 system. These high levels of protein-DNA crosslinking are accompanied by some abnormal replication intermediates.[11] Typically, there are 40S replication intermediates, which may be partially formed and weaker than those caused by DNA polymerase inhibitors, and there are slight accumulations of A- and B-family catenated SV40 chromosomes, indicating inhibition of topoisomerase II-dependent decatenation. The 40S intermediates may indicate that DNA polymerases are being inhibited either directly or indirectly by protein-DNA crosslinks. The signature pattern for direct protein-DNA crosslinking consists of a weak 40S band and slight intensification of catenated dimer bands in association with high levels of protein-DNA crosslinking as measured by the GF/C filter assay (chapter 2).

DNA ALKYLATING AGENTS

Alkylation of DNA may be accompanied by DNA nicking, decreased electrophoretic mobility of the SV40 replication intermediates if the adduct is bulky, and by depurination. The abasic sites resulting from depurination are revealed by alkaline second dimension electrophoresis.[12] Extensive depurination appears to be associated with protein-DNA crosslinking (see discussion in chapter 5). The signature pattern for a bulky DNA alkylating agent such as psorospermin (chapter 5) is shown in Figure 6.1 (Alk).

VALIDATION OF ASSAY

NEGATIVES

A mechanism group-based assay should give no signal for bioactive compounds outside the targeted group. For the SV40 assay, the target group is drugs which disrupt DNA replication. These include both inhibitors of DNA replication enzymes and DNA

damaging agents. Agents outside these groups are uniformly negative for production of aberrant SV40 DNA replication intermediates and for protein crosslinks to replicating viral genomes. A number of purified compounds and plant fractions give no signal in
the SV40 assay, although most of these are cytotoxic. Purified compounds which are negative for disruption of SV40 DNA replication include the microtubule poisons (vinblastine, vincristine,
colchicine), a histone deacetylase inhibitor (sodium butyrate), iono-
phores (monensin, valinomycin, A 23187, nigericin), an inhibitor
of Na^+/K^+ ATPase (ouabain), antimetabolites (methotrexate,
hydroxyurea), polyamine synthesis inhibitors (methylglyoxal
bis[guanylhydrazone], difluoromethyl ornithine) and protein kinase
inhibitors (2-aminopurine, staurosporine). Many of these compounds such as staurosporine, difluoromethyl ornithine and ouabain decrease incorporation of tritiated thymidine into SV40 DNA.
This may be an indication of decreased transport of label or an
indication of nonspecific cytotoxicity due to ion imbalance, unfavorable intracellular pH, ATP depletion, nucleotide precursor pool
imbalance, etc. Since no aberrant replication intermediates or protein-DNA crosslinks are produced, they are treated as negative in
the SV40 assay. Compounds which do not readily cross the cell
membrane, for instance the membrane impermeant protein synthesis inhibitor aurintricarboxylic acid, do not disrupt SV40 DNA
replication in the standard assay. A number of compounds purified on the basis of cytotoxicity against human tumor cells gave
no activity in the SV40 system. These included heymic acid (a
triterpenoid), 2,4-methylene cycloartan-3β-21-diol (a cycloartane
triterpenoid), ethyl linoleate, DM IV (an aliphatic anhydride), DM
IV (Patchouli alcohol), DM VI (an aliphatic ester), MEA II (an
aliphatic acid), oleamide, MEA XXI (an unknown sterol,
MWt = 414, $C_{29}H_{50}O$) and MEA XXII (an unknown alkaloid,
MWt = 346, $C_{16}H_{18}N_4O_5$). The purified polyketides deoxycoriacin
(from *Annona coriaceae*), coriacin (from *Annona coriaceae*) and
annonacin (from *Annona densicoma*) were also negative. It is clear
that many cytotoxic compounds are negative in the SV40 system.
Extremes of pH and temperature have tended to decrease incorporation of label, but have not produced aberrant intermediates or
protein-DNA crosslinks. SV40 DNA replication is insensitive to

charged high molecular weight compounds such as heparin. Tannins were also tested and had no effect on the SV40 DNA replication assay. These high molecular weight polyions can be cytotoxic and, thus, interfere with cytotoxicity assays. They can also interfere with purified enzymes by binding them essentially like ion exchange resins. A number of agents which nick DNA in vitro have also been tested. These were provided by Dr. Linus Shen (Abbott Laboratories) as examples of compounds frequently found in microbial extracts which interfere with in vitro topoisomerase assays. They have no anticancer activity. These compounds were uniformly negative in the SV40 assay. In the SV40 DNA assay, DNA and DNA replication enzymes are shielded from these compounds by the host cell membrane.

Most crude plant fractions are also negative in the SV40 system. None of the fractions derived from black tea by the Kupchan fractionation procedure (see below) showed any activity in the SV40 assay. Caffeine is a weak catalytic inhibitor of topoisomerase II, producing catenated SV40 dimers and acting as an antagonist to topoisomerase II poisons at high concentrations (at the limit of solubility for caffeine).[4] Weak compounds such as caffeine do not give detectable signals in crude extracts. Neither strong perk-brewed coffee nor concentrated instant coffee affected SV40 DNA replication intermediates. It should also be noted that a large number of other compounds have been isolated from coffee, including Ames test mutagens, phenolic compounds, many complex organic acids (feruloylquinic acids up to 2%), mycotoxins, benzo(a)pyrene and other polycyclic aromatic hydrocarbons, complex waxes and oils.[13] Experience with assays on crude plant extracts from the National Cancer Institute's Natural Product Repository has shown that extracts that affect SV40 DNA replication are rare, much less than one percent of the extracts assayed.

From these results, it is clear that SV40 DNA replication is not affected by cytotoxic compounds which do not damage DNA or inhibit DNA replication enzymes. Included in this group are the antimitotics, some investigational drugs and a huge number of cytotoxic compounds without anticancer activity. This latter group includes many natural products which interfere with other drug discovery approaches and necessitate secondary screens and special procedures for their removal. None of these, nor any purified drugs, have caused false positives in the SV40 system. The SV40 system is very sensitive to drugs in four of the mechanistic classes that have consistently produced clinically useful anticancer agents. The freedom from false positives, the ability to screen at very high extract concentrations (3 mg/ml), the detailed mechanistic information provided even at the crude extract level and the economy of the assay all constitute great advantages for a drug discovery approach. The only established, clinically useful group of anticancer drugs not detected is the antimitotics.

NOVEL PATTERNS

Originally, the camptothecin signature was a novel pattern which was not understood. With additional experiments, including two-dimensional neutral-alkaline gel analysis, it was possible to deduce the nature of the aberrant replication intermediates and conclude that they were the result of double strand DNA breaks which occurred at replication forks when they encountered the drug-stabilized topoisomerase I-DNA cleavage complex.[1,14] These double strand DNA breaks are the likely basis for camptothecin's S-phase cytotoxicity.

More recently, psorospermin was found to cause a novel pattern of aberrant SV40 DNA replication intermediates (chapter 5). With additional experiments, it was possible to explain the novel pattern and gain insights into the cytotoxic mechanism of this antileukemic xanthone.[12] These examples show that novel patterns of aberrant SV40 replication intermediates can be analyzed and understood. This is one of the exciting aspects of the SV40 assay system—the potential for discovering drugs which disrupt DNA replication by novel mechanisms.

KNOWN POSITIVE EXTRACT TEST

Crude extracts of *Camptotheca acuminata* leaves, stems and roots (a generous gift from Dr. Randall K. Johnson, SmithKline Beecham Pharmaceuticals) were tested with the SV40 assay. The samples had been extracted with hexane and then with ethyl acetate. A test of an ethyl acetate extract of stems with the SV40 system (3 mg extract per ml of culture medium) showed maximal signals (protein-DNA crosslinks and aberrant intermediates) making up the topoisomerase I poison signature. Experiments were then done over three lower ranges of concentration. The signature patterns were clearly detectable over the entire range from 0.5 µg/ml to 3.0 mg/ml. The protein-DNA crosslinking data are shown in Figure 6.2. The gel patterns for the middle range of concentrations are shown in Figure 6.3. We conclude that an assay at 3 mg extract/ml would be able to detect a camptothecin-like activity at 1/5,000 of the level found in the ethyl acetate extract (0.43% of the ethyl acetate extract dry wt). The ethyl acetate extract of roots had a higher percentage of camptothecin (1.1%). The root extract showed consistently higher levels of protein-DNA crosslinking compared to the stem extract.

The SV40 system is unaffected by most crude extracts and plant fractions. High concentrations of organics alone have no effect on the SV40 system, and screening can be done at very high extract concentrations (> 3 mg/ml) so that minor activities can be detected. Camptothecinoids can be detected by the SV40 system at levels as low as 1/5,000 the levels found in crude extracts of *C. acuminata* stems. Mixing experiments have not yet found a crude extract which can interfere with the detection of camptothecinoids in extracts of *C. acuminata* stems and roots or with the detection of m-AMSA, a topoisomerase II poison. No purified compounds outside the target group, including tannins, have given false positives in the SV40 system. The SV40 assay has been very well validated, and its unique advantages are clear.

DETECTION AND PURIFICATION
OF TOPOISOMERASE II INHIBITORS
USING THE SV40 ASSAY

We have used the SV40 system to examine crude plant extracts for these activities. The plants were extracted and sub-fractionated by the Kupchan procedure.[15] In the Kupchan fractionation procedure, dried plant materials are ground and then extracted by percolation with 95% ethanol at room temperature to give F001. The extracted plant material is dried and repacked for percolation with 50% ethanol, yielding F002. If the material has a high fat content as in the case of seeds, then the ground material is first defatted with hexane (F000) before 95% ethanol percolation. This step minimizes the formation of emulsions between fat and water in subsequent steps. The 95% ethanol fraction (F001) is then partitioned between water and dichloromethane to give fractions F003, F004 and F005. Fraction F004 is further partitioned between hexane and 90% methanol, generating F006 and F007, respectively. Active fractions are further fractionated by chromatography.

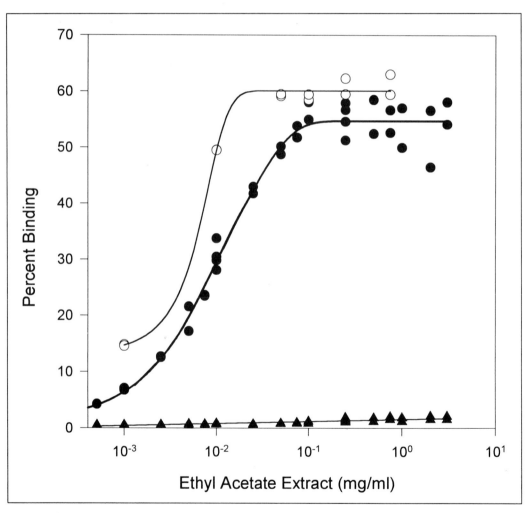

Fig. 6.2. The camptothecin protein-DNA crosslink signal caused by ethyl acetate extracts of C. acuminata *stems and roots over a four order of magnitude concentration range.* ●*, stem extract;* ▲*, stem extract treated with proteinase K before filter assay;* ○*, root extract.*

An early positive in our screen of plants with the SV40 assay was the elephant tree from the Mexican Baja (*Pachycormus discolor*). The crude 95% ethanol extract (Kupchan fraction F001) gave a clear topoisomerase II inhibition signature—increased label in catenated SV40 daughter chromosomes (Fig. 6.4). This same fraction caused low level protein-DNA crosslinking, suggestive of a topoisomerase poison. Subsequent fractionation by the Kupchan procedure gave fractions with increased activity (Fig. 6.5). Both the F004 and F005 fractions were positive for protein-DNA crosslinks and catenation. The specific activity of the F005 fraction was somewhat higher than that of the F004 fraction. However, there was only a slight amount of the F005 compared to F004. Thus, the bulk of the activity was in F004, and this fraction

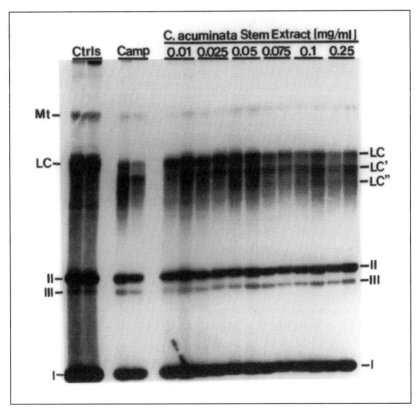

Fig. 6.3. Topoisomerase I poison signature of aberrant SV40 intermediates from ethyl acetate extracts of C. acuminata stems. Abbreviations defined in Figure 6.1.

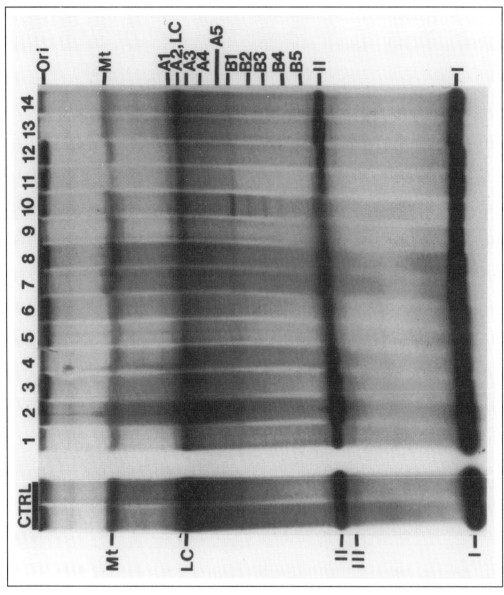

Fig. 6.4. Testing of F001 fractions from 14 plants of the Ohio State University plant collection. Ctrl, controls showing normal SV40 replication intermediates. 1-14, F001 fractions from test plants. Fraction 10 (Pachycormus discolor) shows intense B-family catenated dimer bands, the other samples show only normal replication intermediates. Fraction 10 was also the only one in this set to give protein-DNA crosslinks in the GF/C filter assay. Abbreviations defined in Figure 6.1.

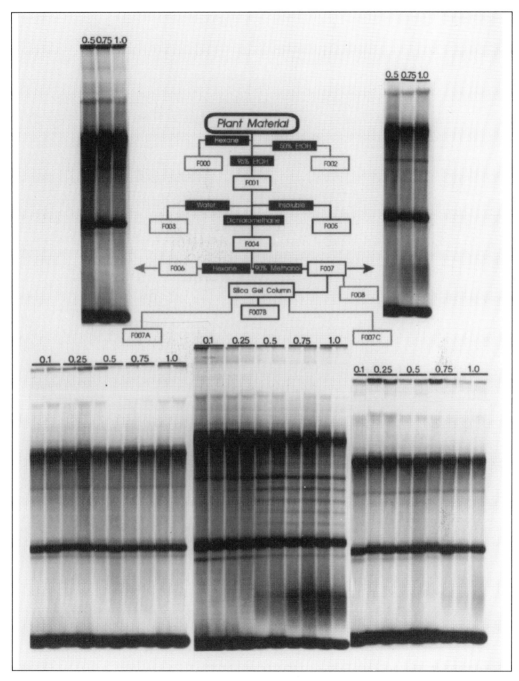

Fig. 6.5. Purification of the Pachycormus discolor *F001 fraction with the Kupchan solvent fractionation scheme and silica gel chromatography. One-dimensional gel analysis of SV40 DNA replication was used to guide the purification. Concentrations are given in mg/ml above each gel lane.*

was used for further purification. A trace of 40S band, indicating replication fork blockage, was also detected in the F004 fraction. The F006 and F008 subfractions were completely inactive. F008 was an insoluble fraction not normally obtained at this step of the Kupchan procedure. The F007 fraction showed catenation, protein-DNA crosslinking and 40S intermediates. The *Pachycormus* F007 fraction was further purified by silica gel chromatography. A column packed with 20 g of dense silica gel was eluted with 50 ml each of seven different solvent mixtures: 100% hexane, 2%, 5%, 10%, 20% and 50% ethyl acetate in hexane, 100% ethyl acetate and 100% methanol. Fractions 29-31, eluted in 50% ethyl acetate in hexane, were pooled as F007A (41.1 mg when dried to powder). Fractions 32-35, eluted in 100% ethyl acetate, were pooled as F007B (172.6 mg). Fractions 36-40, eluted in 100% methanol, were pooled as F007C (91.4 mg). Fraction F007A was inactive, and fraction F007C showed only a trace of 40S intermediates at the highest concentration. In contrast, the F007B fraction showed dose-dependent catenation, protein-DNA crosslinking and 40S structures (Fig. 6.6). This bright yellow material showed several components by thin layer chromatography.

The F007B material was re-chromatographed on another silica gel column to obtain F007B-1, F007B-2 and F007B-3 fractions (Fig. 6.6). F007B-1 showed strong dose-dependent 40S intermediates and weak, but dose-dependent catenation, with protein-DNA crosslinks. The F007B-2 fraction showed a weaker 40S band, and stronger catenation and protein-DNA crosslinking. The F007B-3 fraction showed weak dose-dependent catenation and low protein-DNA crosslinking but no 40S. Thin layer chromatography showed several components in each fraction. The F007B-2 fraction was tested for activity against purified *Drosophila* topoisomerase II (Fig. 6.7). The enzyme was obtained from US Biochemical, and the assay conditions recommended by the supplier were used. The substrate was purified tritium labeled SV40 DNA. Sufficient topoisomerase II was added to give a protein-crosslinking of about five percent. Increasing concentrations of the extract were then added. The total volume of solvent (methanol) was kept constant. This result confirms that the F007B-2 fraction contains a topoisomerase II poison. Following recollection of the plant material, two active compounds (PDB-I and PDB-II) were purified and identified as flavonoids (Fig. 6.8). Members of this group have previously been reported to be topoisomerase II inhibitors and DNA polymerase inhibitors.[16,17] PDB-II, which gave catenated dimers and protein-DNA crosslinks in the SV40 assay, suggesting a topoisomerase II poison, was identified as kaempferol. Kaempferol is a known topoisomerase II poison which fits the structure-activity profile for flavonoid inhibitors of topoisomerase II.[16,17] Kaempferol causes 40S intermediates in SV40 at higher concentrations than those causing topoisomerase II inhibition. These results show that the SV40 system can be used as an assay to detect even weak inhibitors of topoisomerases and DNA polymerases in

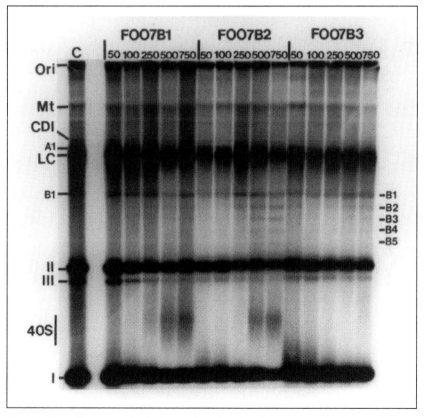

Fig. 6.6. One-dimensional gel electrophoresis of re-chromatographed F007B fraction of Pachycormus discolor. The dose-dependence of catenated dimers and 40S intermediates as a function of extract concentration was tested for each of the three fractions obtained from the re-chromatography.

crude extracts and can guide their purification to homogeneity. The structure-activity profile for inhibition of topoisomerase II by flavonoids is similar to that for inhibition of protein kinase C.[16,17]

Several plant extracts have caused only 40S intermediates in the SV40 assay, indicating DNA polymerase inhibition or

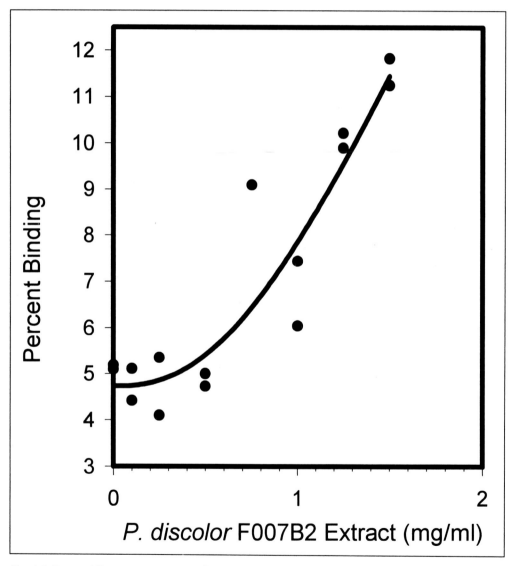

Fig. 6.7. Drosophila *topoisomerase II–dependent protein-DNA crosslinks to purified, tritium-labeled* SV40 DNA *as a function of the concentration of* Pachycormus discolor *F007B2 extract in the assay. This shows that this fraction contains a topoisomerase II poison.*

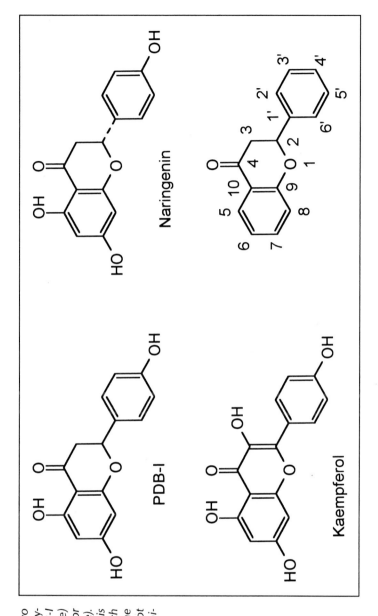

Fig. 6.8. Structures of two active flavonoids of Pachycormus discolor, PDB-I (4',5,7- trihydroxyflavanone) and PDB-II, (kaempferol or 3,4',5,7-tetrahydroxyflavone). The ring numbering system is indicated. Naringenin, which differs from PDB-1 by the stereochemistry at C2, is not a topoisomerase inhibitor.[16,17]

replication fork arrest. A crude (F001) extract of *Polyalthia cerasoides* was a potent inducer of 40S intermediates in one-dimensional gels. The same activity was found in the F003, F006 and F007 Kupchan fractions of this plant. Two-dimensional neutral-chloroquine gel electrophoresis confirmed that the aberrant intermediates seen by one dimensional gel electrophoresis were 40S intermediates (Fig. 6.9). The active compound in *Polyalthia cerasoides* has not yet been purified.

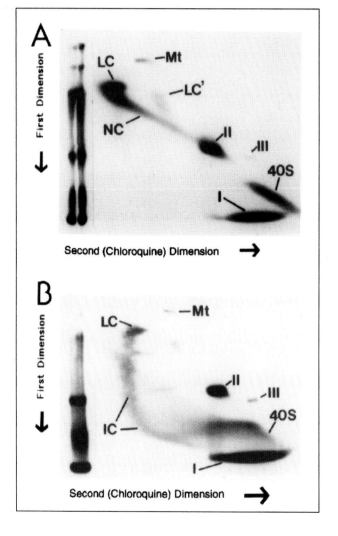

Fig. 6.9. Two-dimensional neutral-chloroquine gel electrophoresis of SV40 DNA replication intermediates produced by aphidicolin and by F001 extract of Polyalthia cerasoides.

REFERENCES

1. Snapka RM. Topoisomerase inhibitors can selectively interfere with different stages of simian virus 40 DNA replication. Mol Cell Biol 1986; 6:4221-4227.

2. Snapka RM, Permana PA, Marquit G et al. Two-dimensional agarose gel analysis of simian virus 40 DNA replication intermediates. Methods: A Companion to Methods in Enzymology 1991; 3:73-82.

3. Shin C-G, Snapka RM. Patterns of strongly protein-associated simian virus 40 DNA replication intermediates resulting from exposures to specific topoisomerase poisons. Biochemistry 1990; 29:10934-10939.

4. Shin C-G, Strayer JM, Wani MA et al. Rapid evaluation of topoisomerase inhibitors: caffeine inhibition of topoisomerases in vivo. Teratogen Carcinogen Mutagen 1990; 10:41-52.

5. Permana PA, Snapka RM, Shen LL et al. Quinobenoxazines: A class of novel antitumor quinolones and potent mammalian DNA topoisomerase II catalytic inhibitors. Biochemistry 1994; 33:11333-11339.

6. Ishida R, Sato M, Narita T et al. Inhibition of DNA topoisomerase II by ICRF-193 induces polyploidization by uncoupling chromosome dynamics from other cell cycle events. J Cell Biol 1994; 126:1341-1351.

7. Chu DTW, Hallas R, Clement JJ et al. Synthesis and antitumor activities of quinolone antineoplastic agents. Drugs Exptl Clin Res 1992; 18:275-282.

8. Elsea SH, Osheroff N, Nitiss JL. Cytotoxicity of quinolones toward eukaryotic cells. Identification of topoisomerase II as the primary cellular target for the quinolone CP-115,953 in yeast. J Biol Chem 1992; 267:13150-13153.

9. Dröge P, Sogo JM, Stahl H. Inhibition of DNA synthesis by aphidicolin induces supercoiling in simian virus 40 replicative intermediates. EMBO J 1985; 4:3241-3246.

10. Snapka RM, Shin C-G, Permana PA et al. Aphidicolin-induced topological and recombinational events in simian virus 40. Nucleic Acids Res 1991; 19:5065-5072.

11. Permana PA, Snapka RM. Aldehyde-induced protein-DNA crosslinks disrupt specific stages of SV40 DNA replication. Carcinogenesis 1994; 15:1031-1036.

12. Permana PA, Ho DK, Cassady JM et al. Mechanism of action of the antileukemic xanthone psorospermin: DNA strand breaks, abasic sites and protein-DNA crosslinks. Cancer Res 1994; 54:3191-3195.

13. Smith RF. New aspects of the chemistry of tea and coffee. III. Zeitschrift für Lebensmittel-Untersuchung und -Forschung 1995; 182:1-7.

14. Shin C-G, Snapka RM. Exposure to camptothecin breaks leading and lagging strand simian virus 40 DNA replication forks. Biochem Biophys Res Commun 1990; 168:135-140.

15. Kupchan SM, Streelman DR, Sneden A. Psorospermin, a new antileukemic xanthone from *Psorospermun febrifugum.* J Natural Prod 1980; 43:296-301.

16. Austin CA, Patel S, Ono K et al. Site-specific DNA cleavage by mammalian DNA topoisomerase II induced by novel flavone and catechin derivatives. Biochem J 1992; 282:883-9.

17. Constantinou A, Mehta R, Runyan C et al. Flavonoids as DNA topoisomerase antagonists and poisons: structure-activity relationships. J Nat Prod 1995; 58:217-225.

CHAPTER 7

SV40 In Vitro DNA Replication: A Potential Model for Studying Anticancer Drug Action

Linda H. Malkas

SV40 is a small DNA tumor virus and a member of the papovavirus family.[1] The viral genome consists of a 5,243 base pair double stranded, covalently closed, circular chromosome. SV40 DNA replication occurs in the nuclei of both monkey and human cells while exhibiting a nonpermissivity for infection in mouse cells. Both the viral chromosome histone composition and its nucleosome structure are essentially identical to that of its host. The initiation of SV40 DNA replication is dependent on only one virally encoded protein, the large T-antigen; all other replication factors are supplied by the permissive host. Replication of the viral DNA is initiated within defined viral sequences known as the origin. Viral DNA replication proceeds bi-directionally and semiconservatively from the origin sequences, terminating about halfway around the molecule from the point of initiation.

The SV40 Replicon Model for Analysis of Anticancer Drugs,
edited by Robert M. Snapka. ©1996 R.G. Landes Company.

An in vitro SV40 DNA replication-elongation system has been described[2] which faithfully completes viral DNA synthesis and chromatin assembly in viral chromosomes that had initiated replication in intact infected cells. In vitro SV40 DNA replication systems have also been developed in which both the initiation and elongation of viral DNA synthesis can be readily studied.[3-7] In these systems purified plasmid DNA containing the SV40 origin, or SV40 chromatin isolated from virus-infected monkey cells, are incubated in soluble extracts prepared from permissive or semi-permissive cells supplemented with purified large T-antigen. Initiation occurs in the defined DNA sequences of the SV40 origin, and the replication reaction proceeds bidirectionally from the origin. The termination of DNA synthesis in the crude extracts occurs as observed in intact cells. The SV40 large T-antigen is the only viral protein required in the in vitro system for the replication of DNA containing the SV40 replication origin. All other factors needed for successful replication are supplied by the host cell extract. Because the viral DNA replication is almost completely dependent on the host cell DNA replication machinery, the in vitro papovavirus DNA replication system is not only invaluable for studying viral DNA synthesis, it is also the best working model currently available for the study of semi-conservative mammalian DNA replication in vitro.

VIRAL COMPONENTS REQUIRED FOR SV40 IN VITRO DNA REPLICATION

The DNA sequences in the SV40 origin that are essential for SV40 DNA replication have been defined in vivo[8-15] and shown to be the same for in vitro viral DNA synthesis.[5,16,17] The DNA sequence domains defined as the minimal core origin for SV40 DNA replication include the inverted GAGGC repeat in the large T-antigen binding site I, the large T-antigen binding site II, and the A-T rich region on the late transcription side of the origin.[16,18] Additionally, it was demonstrated by Li et al[16] that, although the entire large T-antigen binding site I[19] was not required for DNA replication, its presence increased the efficiency of replication both in vitro and in intact cells. Furthermore, the SP1 binding sites[20,21] and the SV40 72 base pair repeat enhancer sequences[12,22] were shown to have little effect on replication in vitro, though the presence of either element increased the level of replication in intact cells.[16]

The only other viral component required for in vitro SV40 DNA replication, besides the minimal core SV40 origin, is the SV40 encoded large T-antigen.[4] The large T-antigen is a multifunctional phosphoprotein, M_r 94,000, having the ability to specifically bind DNA sequences in the SV40 origin; it possesses an ATPase activity, and it can form complexes with both the cellular p53[1] and retinoblastoma (Rb) proteins.[23]

The ability to readily purify a homogenous SV40 large T-antigen from infected cells by immunoaffinity chromatography[24,25] has permitted some insight into this protein's role in the initiation and possibly the elongation phase of SV40 DNA synthesis. It has been demonstrated that the large T-antigen has an associated DNA helicase activity.[26] This DNA helicase activity was shown to be inhibited by several large T-antigen specific monoclonal antibodies suggesting that the activity is intrinsic to the large T-antigen protein. Additionally, it was demonstrated that mutant large T-antigen proteins, defective in ATPase function, also exhibit decreased DNA helicase activity.[26] The role played by large T-antigen in the initiation of in vitro SV40 DNA replication has recently been reviewed.[27,28] Briefly, the large T-antigen binds to specific sites within the SV40 origin and melts the early palindrome region within the origin region. The addition of topoisomerase I and RP-A (two mammalian cell proteins that function in DNA synthesis and which will be described later in this chapter) facilitates the further melting of the SV40 DNA, presumably allowing access of other DNA replication proteins to the DNA.

MAMMALIAN CELL PROTEINS REQUIRED FOR THE EFFICIENT REPLICATION OF SV40 ORIGIN CONTAINING DNA IN VITRO

The employment of the SV40-based cell-free DNA replication systems has identified several mammalian enzymes and proteins required for DNA synthesis in vitro (reviewed in refs. 29-33).

A variety of evidence indicates that DNA polymerase is a major replicative polymerase in intact eukaryotic cells (reviewed in refs. 34, 35). That DNA polymerase also played a role in in vitro SV40 DNA replication was suggested when it was observed that the in vitro DNA synthesis in crude cell extracts was readily inhibited by aphidicolin.[4-7] The absolute requirement for DNA polymerase α, and its tightly associated DNA primase, in the initiation events of in vitro SV40 DNA synthesis has been shown by the work of Wobbe et al,[36] Wold et al,[37] Tsurimoto et al,[38] Weinberg et al,[39] Collins and Kelly[40] and Denis and Bullock[41] using reconstituted DNA replication systems. Several studies suggest that DNA polymerase α-primase may also specifically interact with the SV40 large T-antigen to facilitate the initiation of DNA synthesis.[40,42-45]

DNA polymerase δ[46,47] has also been shown to have a role in the synthesis of SV40 replication origin containing DNA in vitro.[48,49] It has been suggested that the DNA polymerases α and δ function synchronously during DNA synthesis.[49-53] Models have been suggested for the coordinated function of the DNA polymerases in SV40 in vitro DNA replication.[31,38,50,52,53] In one model, DNA polymerase α-primase mediates replication initiation events as well as the synthesis of the lagging strand DNA during chain elongation.[31,38,50,52] DNA polymerase δ is envisioned in this model as conducting leading strand synthesis during DNA chain elongation.[31,38,50,52] In another recently proposed model, DNA polymerase α-primase functions in the synthesis of primers for the initiation of in vitro DNA synthesis at the SV40 origin and in the priming of each new Okazaki fragment during DNA replication. In this model it is DNA polymerase δ that is responsible for replicating both daughter strands in vitro.[53]

A protein complex designated RF-C[50] or A1[51] has also been reported to be important for the efficient in vitro replication of DNA containing the SV40 origin. Results reported by Tsurimoto and Stillman[50,52] and Waga and Stillman[53] suggest that RF-C facilitates the coordinated synthesis of both the leading and lagging strands during DNA replication. These researchers suggest that RF-C may act as a connector or hinge between the DNA polymerases α and δ.

Another cellular factor suggested by the current evidence to be involved in in vitro SV40 replication has been purified and identified as the proliferating cell nuclear antigen, PCNA.[48,54] This protein stimulates the processivity of DNA polymerase δ and has been designated as an auxiliary factor for the polymerase.[55-57] PCNA's role in replication has been implicated by its ability to greatly stimulate in vitro SV40 DNA synthesis.[48,58,59] Due to PCNA's interaction with DNA polymerase δ the protein is envisioned to act at the elongation phase of DNA replication.

A cellular derived single stranded DNA binding protein (SSB) has a role in stabilizing the newly formed single stranded regions created in replicating DNA by the helicase activity of the large T-antigen.[36,37,60] It was observed that the presence of the SV40 origin sequence in duplex DNA and a single strand DNA binding protein appeared to be the only requirements for the SV40 large T-antigen to catalyze the unwinding reaction. A protein that functions as a eukaryotic single strand DNA binding protein has been purified to apparent homogeneity from HeLa cells[37] and human 293 cells.[61] The isolated protein, which has been designated by various laboratories as RP-A, RF-A or HSSB, is a multi-subunit protein containing three associated polypeptides of 70, 32-34, and 11-14 kDa. The single stranded DNA binding proteins purified from species other than human or yeast were observed to inhibit DNA polymerase α-primase activity but not DNA polymerase δ activity.[62] The isolated human cell protein binds single stranded DNA and is required for the large T-antigen mediated unwinding of duplex DNA molecules containing the SV40 origin.

In intact cells SV40 uses host DNA topoisomerases for viral DNA replication.[63-69] DNA topoisomerases I and II have also been suggested to play a role in in vitro SV40 DNA replication by Yang et al.[70] These workers were able to restore in vitro SV40 DNA replication activity by adding purified topoisomerases I and II to depleted cell extracts. In addition, it was observed that either the topoisomerase I or II enzyme could carry out the unwinding activity required for the progression of the replication fork. However, a unique role was also described for topoisomerase II in SV40 DNA synthesis in vitro. It was observed that topoisomerase II can also function in the segregation of newly replicated daughter molecules.[70]

A MULTIPROTEIN FORM OF DNA POLYMERASE MEDIATES PAPOVAVIRUS DNA REPLICATION IN VITRO

Although human cell derived DNA polymerases α and δ, RP-A, RF-C, topoisomerases I and II, and PCNA have been identified as playing a role in SV40 DNA replication in vitro, their functional organization allowing for the efficient replication of DNA has not been well defined. Evidence for multiprotein complexes playing a role in DNA replication has grown over the years (reviewed in refs. 32, 34, 71, 72). We have previously reported on a replication-competent multiprotein form of DNA polymerase isolated from human (HeLa) cell extracts that was observed to sediment at 18-21S during velocity sedimentation analyses.[73-75,99] The proteins found to co-purify with the human cell multiprotein form of DNA polymerase include: DNA polymerase α, DNA primase, topoisomerase I, PCNA,[75] DNA polymerase δ, topoisomerase II, DNA helicase, DNA ligase I and RF-C.[99] The multiprotein form of the human cell DNA polymerase was further purified by Q-Sepharose chromatography and shown to be fully competent for supporting origin-specific and large-T-antigen-dependent in vitro SV40 DNA replication.[75] In addition, measurable replication activity by the human cell multiprotein form of DNA polymerase depends on in vitro assay requirements[99] that are comparable to those observed in intact cells[1] and with crude extracts prepared from cells that are permissive for viral DNA synthesis.[4,5,7,36]

This laboratory has also recently identified and characterized a 17S multiprotein form of DNA polymerase from murine (FM3A) cells[76] that is capable of supporting DNA replication using another papovavirus (the polyomavirus) based in vitro DNA synthesis system.[77,78] Polyomavirus in vitro DNA synthesis, like that of SV40, is dependent on the polyoma viral large T-antigen, viral origin sequences and DNA replication factors isolated from permissive (mouse) cells. The proteins and enzymatic activities identified to co-purify with the mouse cell multiprotein form of DNA polymerase include: DNA polymerases α and δ, DNA primase, PCNA, DNA ligase I, DNA helicase, and DNA topoisomerases I and II. It was also demonstrated that the integrity of the murine cell multiprotein form of DNA polymerase was maintained after treatment with detergents, salt, RNase or DNase, suggesting that the association of the proteins with one another was independent of nonspecific interactions with other cellular macromolecular components. It was proposed that the isolated mouse cell multiprotein form of DNA polymerase represented a mammalian Multiprotein DNA Replication Complex (MRC). We introduced a model to represent the mouse cell MRC based on the fractionation and chromatographic profiles of the individual proteins found to co-purify with the complex.[76] The proposed model for the MRC was recently extended to include the human cell multiprotein form of DNA polymerase.[99]

ANTICANCER DRUG ACTION ON IN VITRO SV40 DNA REPLICATION ACTIVITY IN CRUDE CELL EXTRACTS

Due to the limitations of most of the anticancer chemotherapeutics available today a considerable effort is being made to discover more effective and discriminating anticancer drugs. Paralleling this effort is the need for developing rapid, accurate, and reliable methods for evaluating the usefulness of these new compounds, and describing their potential mechanisms of action.

One approach that has been employed in an attempt to determine whether a potential chemotherapeutic agent directly affects cellular DNA synthesis has been the use of individual DNA replication enzymes that have been purified from animal cells. This method evaluates whether the anticancer agent affects the activity of a particular, isolated DNA replication protein. The results are then extrapolated to predict whether the agent potentially affects cellular DNA synthesis. Testing whether the activity of individually purified DNA replication proteins can be affected by anticancer agents has produced some successes in defining the potential mechanism of action of several drugs (for examples see Furth and Cohen,[79] Momparler,[80] Hsiang et al,[81] Rowe et al,[82] Ohno et al,[83] Hsiang and Liu,[66] Mikita and Beardsley,[84] Kawato et al,[85] Kuchta and Willhelm,[86] Perrino and Mekosh,[87] Bachur et al,[88,89] Huang et al[90]). However, several limitations must also be considered while using individually isolated DNA replication proteins when attempting to either screen for potential anticancer agents or infer the mechanism of action of a drug that affects cellular DNA synthesis.

First, there are a number of proteins involved in the DNA synthetic process in intact cells, and each would need to be individually purified and tested in order to conduct a screen for new agents. Second, not all of the enzymes and proteins involved in mammalian cell DNA replication have been identified, so the target-protein activity of a given anticancer drug could be missing from the current panel of known DNA replication proteins. And third, the interaction of an anticancer drug with its "target-protein" may be quite different when this protein is itself interacting with other cellular components, as opposed to when this protein is acting alone in the presence of the drug. Some of these concerns regarding the use of isolated enzymes to describe a drug's mechanism of action are supported by published reports in which the concentration of an anticancer drug that is needed to inhibit the activity of a given purified protein greatly exceeds that required to promote cellular cytotoxicity (for examples see Kufe and Major,[91] Glisson et al[92]).

Recently, there have been efforts made to employ in vitro SV40 DNA replication as a potential model for evaluating anticancer drug action. The strengths of this model for studying drug action include: (1) that it can mediate various aspects of the DNA replication process; (2) that it permits the accurate assessment of whether an anticancer chemotherapeutic drug has the ability to directly interact with the DNA synthetic process while being uncoupled from any other cellular processes that may secondarily affect DNA synthesis; and (3) it would permit the investigator to examine the anticancer drug's ability to affect the entire DNA replication apparatus, and not only isolated individual protein components which have a role in the DNA synthetic process.

Several studies evaluating anticancer drug effects on the in vitro SV40 DNA replication activity in crude HeLa extracts have been reported. Camptothecin (CPT), an inhibitor of topoisomerase I,[81] was observed to slightly reduce the level of SV40 DNA replication in a crude cell extract.[70] These workers also reported that epipodophyllotoxin (VM-26), an inhibitor of topoisomerase II,[93] profoundly altered the types of SV40 in vitro DNA replication products normally produced in crude extracts. Ishimi et al[94] performed studies to examine the effect of a novel topoisomerase II inhibitor, ICRF-193, on crude HeLa extract in vitro SV40 DNA replication activity. These workers used as the parental DNA template either a plasmid DNA containing the SV40 origin of replication or SV40 chromosomes, prepared from infected cells. Their results suggest that ICRF-193 inhibits both the decatenation of intertwined daughter dimer molecules and the unwinding of the terminal region of the parental DNA, during the late stage of SV40 DNA replication in vitro. However, ICRF-193 was observed to completely inhibit late stage in vitro DNA synthesis of the purified SV40 chromosomes. These findings are consistent with previously reported results indicating that topoisomerase II is required for unwinding of the final duplex DNA in the late stage of SV40 chromosome replication in vitro in crude cell extracts.[70]

The SV40 in vitro DNA synthesis system was also used to evaluate the interaction between replication forks and topoisomerase I-CPT-DNA ternary cleavable complexes.[95] The formation of topoisomerase I-CPT-DNA cleavable complexes on plasmid DNA containing the SV40 origin profoundly and irreversibly inhibited SV40 in vitro DNA replication. Aberrant types of DNA replication products were formed whose relative abundance varied with the concentrations of exogenously added topoisomerase I and CPT. Analysis of the aberrant replication products suggested what the authors called a "collision" model for the interaction between the advancing DNA replication fork and a topoisomerase I-CPT-DNA cleavable complex. The "collision" would result in an irreversible arrest of replication fork movement and the formation of a double strand DNA break at the fork. Concomitant with the DNA fork arrest and breakage, the reversible cleavable complex would be converted into a topoisomerase I-linked DNA break. These authors' findings and the suggested "collision" model are consistent with previously reported results and proposed models for the action of CPT at DNA replication forks in intact cells.[63-65,68,96]

ANTICANCER DRUG ACTION ON IN VITRO SV40 DNA SYNTHESIS MEDIATED BY A MULTIPROTEIN FORM OF DNA POLYMERASE

We have initiated studies to evaluate the potential of the replication-competent multiprotein form of DNA polymerase (MRC)[75,76] to serve as a model for studying anticancer drug action.

We selected clinically relevant anticancer drugs that are known to inhibit the S-phase of the animal cell cycle, to serve as representative chemotherapeutics in order to evaluate the MRC model system for the study of anti-neoplastic agents that directly affect mammalian cell DNA replication. The anticancer agents chosen for these studies were: ara-CTP, the active metabolite of ara-C,[97,98] etoposide (VP-16),[93] and camptothecin.[81] In these experiments, we determined whether the concentrations of CPT, VP-16 and ara-C (ara-CTP) that effectively inhibited HeLa intact cell DNA synthesis also interfered with the ability of the MRC, derived from HeLa cells,[75] to support in vitro SV40 DNA replication. For these studies, drug dose-response curves were prepared to assess the degree of inhibition of MRC-mediated DNA replication as a function of anticancer agent concentration. IC_{50} values for the inhibition of MRC-mediated in vitro SV40 DNA replication were determined for each anticancer agent from these dose response curves (Table 7.1). The IC_{50} for the inhibition of intact HeLa cell DNA synthesis was also determined for each of these anticancer agents (Table 7.1).

The IC_{50} values derived for the inhibition of MRC-mediated in vitro SV40 DNA replication are comparable to those determined for intact HeLa cell DNA synthesis (Table 7.1). These results suggest that the in vitro SV40 DNA replication model system utilizing the HeLa cell MRC may serve as an accurate representation of the cellular DNA replication machinery, and thus be useful for the analysis of anticancer agents that directly affect cellular DNA synthesis.

PERSPECTIVE

Some of the limitations currently associated with anticancer chemotherapy are due in part to the slow empirical basis in which many of the clinical regimens are developed. A consequence of this approach has been that a significant lag time occurs between the accumulation of evidence for anticancer activity of an antitumor agent, its introduction into clinical use, and the definition of its mechanism of action. Therefore there is currently a need for developing rapid, accurate and reliable methods for evaluating the usefulness of potential anticancer agents and for describing their mechanism of action. The recent studies utilizing in vitro SV40 DNA replication as a model system for evaluating anticancer drug action suggest that this model may be especially useful in clarifying possible mechanisms by which these drugs affect the DNA replication process. The true power of the in vitro SV40 DNA replication model system for investigating the mechanism of action of anticancer drugs that directly affect cellular DNA synthesis should be realized in the next few years.

Table 7.1. Anticancer drug IC_{50} values for MRC-mediated SV40 DNA replication activity and intact HeLa cell DNA synthesis

IC_{50} for in vitro MRC replication activity[a] synthesis[b]		IC_{50} for HeLa cell DNA
ARA-CTP		**ARA-C**
	50 nM	80 nM
Camptothecin		**Campothecin**
	0.5 μM	1 μM
Etoposide		**Etoposide**
	5 μM	10 μM

[a] The HeLa cell MRC was prepared as described in ref. 75. MRC-mediated in vitro DNA replication assays were performed as described[75] in the absence or the presence of a range of concentrations of ara-CTP, camptothecin (CPT), and etoposide (VP-16). Dimethylsulfonyl oxide (DMSO) serves as the solvent for stock solutions of VP-16 and CPT. Control reactions were performed to assay for the effects of DMSO on MRC-mediated DNA replication. Drug dose-response curves for ara-CTP, CPT and VP-16 were prepared by plotting the number of nanomoles of ^{32}P-TTP incorporated into SV40-origin containing plasmid DNA during DNA replication reactions carried out by the MRC at each drug concentration chosen. IC_{50} values of the MRC's DNA synthetic activity were determined from these drug dose-response curves.
[b] Exponentially growing HeLa cells, on 60 mm tissue culture plates (5 x 10^4 cells/plate), were incubated for 1hr at 37°C with varying concentrations of ara-C, CPT, or VP-16 in the presence of ^{3}H-thymidine incorporation into DNA molecules. Drug dose-response curves for the inhibition of intact HeLa cell DNA synthesis by ara-C, CPT, or VP-16 were prepared by plotting drug concentration versus number of nanomoles of ^{3}H-thymidine incorporated into cellular DNA (per plate). The IC_{50} values for ara-C, CPT, and VP-16 inhibition of HeLa cell DNA synthesis were deduced from these dose-response curves.

ACKNOWLEDGMENTS

The author would like to thank the members of her laboratory, especially Jennifer Coll, Philip Wills, and Yuetong Wei for their preparation of the data that are represented in Table 7.1. The author would also like to thank Dr. Robert J. Hickey for his reading and comments regarding this manuscript, and Ms. Evelyn Elizabeth for the typing of this manuscript.

The experimental results described from the author's laboratory were supported by awards from the National Institutes of Health/National Cancer Institute and the Maryland Designated Research Initiative Foundation made to LHM.

REFERENCES

1. DePamphilis ML, Bradley MK. Replication of SV40 and polyoma virus chromosomes. In: Salzman NP, ed. The Papovaviridae Volume I: The Polyomaviruses. New York: Plenum Press 1986:99-246.
2. DePamphilis ML, Wassarman PM. Replication of eukaryotic chromosomes: a close-up of the replication fork. Ann Rev Biochem 1982; 49:627-666.
3. Ariga H, Sugano S. Initiation of simian virus 40 DNA replication in vitro. J Virol 1983; 48:481-491.
4. Li JJ, Kelly TJ. Simian virus 40 DNA replication in vitro. Proc Natl Acad Sci USA 1984; 81:6973-6977.
5. Stillman B, Gluzman Y. Replication and supercoiling of simian virus 40 DNA in cell extracts from human cells. Mol Cell Biol 1985; 5:2051-2060.
6. Wobbe CR, Dean F, Weissbach L et al. In vitro replication of duplex circular DNA containing the simian virus 40 DNA origin site. Proc Acad Sci USA 1985; 82:5710-5714.
7. Decker RS, Yamaguchi M, Possenti R et al. In vitro initiation of DNA replication in SV40 chromosomes. J Biol Chem 1987; 262:10863-10872.
8. Subramanian KN, Shenk T. Definition of the boundaries of the origin of DNA replication in simian virus 40. Nucleic Acids Res 1978; 5:3635-3640.
9. Shortle D, Nathans D. Regulatory mutants of simian virus 40: constructed mutants with base substitutions at the origin of DNA replication. J Mol Biol 1979; 131:801-808.
10. DiMaio D, Nathans D. Cold-sensitive regulatory mutants of simian virus 40. J Mol Biol 1980; 140:129-142.

11. Myers RM, Tjian R. Construction and analysis of SV40 origins defective in tumor antigen binding and DNA replication. Proc Natl Acad Sci USA 1980; 77:6491-6495.

12. Fromm M, Berg P. Deletion mapping of DNA regions required for SV40 early region promoter function in vivo. J Mol Appl Genet 1982; 1:457-481.

13. Bergsma DJ, Olive DM, Hartzell SW et al. Territorial limits and functional anatomy of the simian virus 40 replication origin. Proc Natl Acad Sci USA 1982; 79:381-385.

14. Jones KA, Myers RM, Tjian R. Mutational analysis of simian virus 40 large T-antigen DNA binding sites. EMBO J 1984; 3:3247-3255.

15. Hertz GZ, Young MR, Mertz JE. The A+T-rich sequence of the simian virus 40 origin is essential for replication and is involved in bending of the viral DNA. J Virol 1987; 61:2322-2325.

16. Li JJ, Peden KWC, Dixon RAF et al. Functional organization of the simian virus 40 origin of DNA replication. Mol Cell Biol 1986; 6:1117-1128.

17. Deb S, DeLucia AL, Koff A et al. The adenine-thymine domain of the simian virus 40 core origin directs DNA bending and coordinately regulates DNA replication. Mol Cell Biol 1986; 6:4578-4584.

18. Stillman B, Gerard RD, Guggenheimer RA et al. T-antigen and template requirements for SV40 DNA replication in vitro. EMBO J 1985; 4:2933-2939.

19. Tjian R. Protein-DNA interactions at the origin of simian virus 40 DNA replication. Cold Spring Harbor Symp Quant Biol 1978; 43:655-662.

20. Dynan WS, Tjian R. The promoter specific transcription factor Sp1 binds to upstream sequences in the SV40 early promoter. Cell 1983; 35:79-87.

21. Gidoni D, Dynan WS, Tjian R. Multiple specific contacts between a mammalian transcription factor and its cognate promoters. Nature 1984; 312:409-413.

22. Moreau P, Hen R, Wasylyk B et al. The SV40 72 base pair repeat has a striking effect on gene expression both in SV40 and other chimeric recombinants. Nucleic Acids Res 1981; 9:6047-6068.

23. DeCaprio JA, Ludlow JW, Figge J et al. SV40 large T-antigen forms a specific complex with the product of the retinoblastoma susceptibility gene. Cell 1988; 54:275-283.

24. Simanis V, Lane DP. An immunoaffinity purification procedure for SV40 large T antigen. Virol 1985; 144:88-100.

25. Dixon RAF, Nathans D. Purification of simian virus 40 large T antigen by immunoaffinity chromatography. J Virol 1985; 53:1001-1004.

26. Stahl H, Droge P, Knippers R. DNA helicase activity of SV40 large tumor antigen. EMBO J 1986; 5:1939-1944.

27. Borowiec JA, Dean FB, Bullock PA et al. Binding and unwinding—How T antigen engages the SV40 origin of DNA replication. Cell 1990; 60:181-184.

28. Fanning E, Knippers R. Structure and function of simian virus 40 large tumor antigen. Ann Rev Biochem 1992; 61:55-85.

29. Challberg M, Kelly T. Animal virus DNA replication. Ann Rev Biochem 1989; 58:671-717.

30. Stillman B. Initiation of eukaryotic DNA replication in vitro. Ann Rev Cell Biol 1989; 5:197-245.

31. Hurwitz J, Dean FB, Kwong AD et al. The in vitro replication of DNA containing the SV40 origin. J Biol Chem 1990; 265: 18043-18046.

32. Malkas LH, Hickey RJ, Baril EF. Multienzyme complexes for DNA synthesis in eukaryotes: P-4 revisited. In: Strauss PR, Wilson SH, ed(s). Molecular Biochemistry and Macromolecular Assemblies. New Jersey: The Telford Press 1990:45-68.

33. Stillman B, Bell SP, Dutta A et al. In: Regulation of the Eukaryotic Cell Cycle. Chichester: John Wiley & Sons, 1992:147-156.

34. Fry M, Loeb LA. Animal cell DNA polymerases. Boca Raton, Fl: CRC Press, Inc 1986.

35. Burgers PMJ. Eukaryotic DNA polymerase α and δ: conserved properties and interactions, from yeast to mammalian cells. Prog Nucleic Acid Res 1989; 37:235-280.

36. Wobbe CR, Weissbach L, Borowiec JA et al. Replication of simian virus 40 origin-containing DNA in vitro with purified proteins. Proc Natl Acad Sci USA 1987; 84:1834-1838.

37. Wold MS, Kelly TJ. Purification and characterization of replication protein A, a cellular protein required for in vitro replication of simian virus 40 DNA. Proc Natl Acad Sci USA 1988; 85:2523-2527.

38. Tsurimoto T, Melendy T, Stillman B. Sequential initiation of lagging and leading strand synthesis by two different polymerase complexes at the SV40 DNA replication origin. Nature 1990; 346:534-539.

39. Weinberg DH, Collins KL, Simancek P et al. Reconstitution of SV40 DNA replication with purified proteins. Proc Natl Acad Sci USA 1990; 87:8692-8696.

40. Collins KL, Kelly TJ. Effects of T antigen and replication protein A on the initiation of DNA synthesis by DNA polymerase α-primase. Mol Cell Biol 1991; 11:2108-2115.

41. Denis D, Bullock PA. Primer-DNA formation during simian virus 40 DNA replication in vitro. Mol Cell Biol 1993; 13:2882-2890.

42. Smale S, Tjian R. T-antigen-simian virus 40 DNA polymerase complex implicated in simian virus 40 DNA replication. Mol Cell Biol 1986; 6:4077-4087.

43. Gannon JV, Lane DP. p53 and DNA polymerase alpha compete for binding to SV40 T antigen. Nature 1987; 329:456-458.

44. Dornreiter I, Höss A, Arthur AK et al. SV40 T antigen binds directly to the large subunit of purified DNA polymerase alpha. EMBO J 1990; 9:3329-3336.

45. Gannon JV, Lane DP. Interactions between SV40 T antigen and DNA polymerase α. New Biol 1990; 2:84-92.

46. Byrnes JJ, Downey KM, Black VL et al. A new mammalian DNA polymerase with 3' to 5' exonuclease activity: DNA polymerase δ. Biochem 1976; 15:2817-2823.

47. Lee MYWT, Tan C-K, Downey KM et al. Further studies on calf thymus DNA polymerase δ purified to homogeneity by a new procedure. Biochem 1984; 23:1906-1913.

48. Prelich G, Tan C-K, Mikostura M et al. Functional identity of proliferating cell nuclear antigen and a DNA polymerase-δ auxiliary protein. Nature 1987; 326:517-520.

49. Melendy T, Stillman B. Purification of DNA polymerase δ as an essential simian virus 40 DNA replication factor. J Biol Chem 1991; 266:1942-1949.

50. Tsurimoto T, Stillman B. Multiple replication factors augment DNA synthesis by the two eukaryotic DNA polymerases, α and δ. EMBO J 1989; 8:3883-3889.

51. Lee S-H, Eki T, Hurwitz J. Synthesis of DNA containing the simian virus 40 origin of replication by the combined action of DNA polymerases α and δ. Proc Natl Acad Sci USA 1989; 86:7361-7365.

52. Tsurimoto T, Stillman B. Replication factors required for SV40 DNA replication in vitro. J Biol Chem 1991; 266:1961-1968.

53. Waga S, Stillman B. Anatomy of a DNA replication fork revealed by reconstitution of SV40 DNA replication in vitro. Nature 1994; 369:207-212.

54. Wold MS, Weinberg DH, Virshup DM et al. Identification of cellular proteins required for simian virus 40 DNA replication. J Biol Chem 1989; 264:2801-2809.

55. Tan CK, Castillo C, So AG et al. An auxiliary protein for DNA polymerase-δ from fetal calf thymus. J Biol Chem 1986; 261:12310-12316.

56. Bravo R, Frank R, Blundell PA et al. Cyclin/PCNA is the auxiliary protein of DNA polymerase δ. Nature 1987; 326:515-517.

57. Downey KM, Tan CK, Andrews DMM et al. Proposed roles for DNA polymerase alpha and delta at the replication fork. Cancer Cells 1988; 6:1211-1218.

58. Prelich G, Stillman B. Coordinated leading and lagging strand synthesis during SV40 DNA replication in vitro requires PCNA. Cell 1988; 53:117-126.

59. Wold MS, Li JJ, Kelly TJ. Initiation of simian virus 40 DNA replication in vitro: large-tumor-antigen and origin-dependent unwinding of the template. Proc Natl Acad Sci USA 1987; 84:3643-3647.

60. Dodson M, Dean FB, Bullock P et al. Unwinding of duplex DNA from the SV40 origin of replication by T antigen. Science 1987; 238:964-967.

61. Fairman MP, Stillman B. Cellular factors required for multiple stages of SV40 DNA replication in vitro. EMBO J 1988; 7:1211-1218.

62. Kenny MK, Lee S-H, Hurwitz J. Multiple functions of human single stranded-DNA binding protein in simian virus 40 DNA replication: Single strand stabilization and stimulation of DNA polymerases α and δ. Proc Natl Acad Sci USA 1989; 86:9757-9761.

63. Snapka RM. Topoisomerase inhibitors can selectively interfere with different stages of simian virus 40 DNA replication. Mol Cell Biol 1986; 6:4221-4227.

64. Snapka RM, Powelson MA, Strayer JM. Swiveling and decatenation of replicating simian virus 40 genomes in vivo. Mol Cell Biol 1988; 8:515-521.

65. Avemann K, Knippers R, Koller T et al. Camptothecin, a specific inhibitor of type I DNA topoisomerase, induces DNA breakage at replication forks. Mol Cell Biol 1988; 8:3026-3034.

66. Hsiang Y-H, Liu LF. Identification of mammalian DNA topoisomerase I as an intracellular target of the anticancer drug camptothecin. Cancer Res 1988; 48:1722-1726.

67. Porter SE, Champoux JJ. Mapping in vivo topoisomerase I sites on simian virus 40 DNA: asymmetric distribution of sites on replicating molecules. Mol Cell Biol 1989; 9:541-550.

68. Shin C-G, Snapka RM. Exposure to camptothecin breaks leading and lagging strand simian virus 40 DNA replication forks. Biochem Biophys Res Commun 1990; 168:135-140.

69. Parker LH, Champoux JJ. Analysis of the biased distribution of topoisomerase I break sites on replicating simian virus 40 DNA. J Mol Biol 1993; 231:6-18.

70. Yang L, Wold MS, Li JJ et al. Roles of DNA topoisomerases in simian virus 40 DNA replication in vitro. Proc Natl Acad Sci USA 1987; 84:950-954.

71. Mathews CK, Slabaugh MB. Eukaryotic DNA metabolism. Are deoxynucleotides channeled to replication sites? Exp Cell Res 1986; 162:285-295.

72. Reddy G, Fager R. Replitase: a complex integrating dNTP synthesis and DNA replication. Crit Rev Eukaryotic Gene Exp 1993; 3:255-277.

73. Hickey RJ, Malkas LH, Pedersen N et al. Multienzyme complex for DNA replication in HeLa cells. In: Moses R, Summers W, eds. DNA Replication and Mutagenesis. Washington, DC: Amer Soc Microbiol 1988:41-54.

74. Baril EF, Malkas LH, Hickey RJ et al. A multiprotein DNA polymerase α complex from HeLa cells: interaction with other proteins in DNA replication. Cancer Cells 1988; 6:373-384.

75. Malkas LH, Hickey RJ, Li C et al. A 21S enzyme complex from HeLa cells that functions in simian virus 40 DNA replication in vitro. Biochem 1990; 29:6362-6374.

76. Wu Y, Hickey R, Lawlor K et al. A 17S form of DNA polymerase from mouse cells mediates the in vitro replication of polyomavirus DNA. J Cell Biochem 1994; 54:32-46.

77. Murakami Y, Eki T, Yamada M et al. Species-specific in vitro synthesis of DNA containing the polyomavirus origin of replication. Proc Natl Acad Sci USA 1986; 83:6347-6351.

78. Dermody JJ, Lawlor KG, Du H et al. Polyomavirus DNA sythesis in vitro: studies with CHO, 3T3 and their tsDNA mutants. Cancer Cells 1988; 6:95-100.

79. Furth JJ, Cohen SS. Inhibition of mammalian DNA polymerase by the 5'-triphosphate of 1-β-D arabinofuranosylcytosine and the 5'-triphosphate of 1-β-D arabinofuranosyladenine. Cancer Res 1968; 28:2061-2067.

80. Momparler R. Effect of cytosine arabinoside 5'-triphosphate on mammalian DNA polymerase. Biochem Biophys Res Commun 1969; 34:465-471.

81. Hsiang Y-H, Hertzberg R, Hecht S et al. Camptothecin induces protein-linked DNA breaks via mammalian DNA topoisomerase I. J Biol Chem 1985; 260:14873-14878.

82. Rowe TC, Chen GL, Hsiang Y-H et al. DNA damage by antitumor acridines mediated by mammalian DNA topoisomerase II. Cancer Res 1986; 46:2021-2026.

83. Ohno Y, Spriggs D, Matsukage A et al. Effects of 1-β-D arabinofuranosylcytosine incorporation on elongation of specific DNA sequences by DNA polymerase β. Cancer Res 1988; 48:1494-1498.

84. Mikita T, Beardsley GP. Functional consequences of the arabinosylcytosine structural lesions in DNA. Biochem 1988; 27: 4698-4705.

85. Kawato Y, Aonuma M, Hirota Y et al. Intracellular roles of SN-38, a metabolite of the camptothecin derivative CPT-11, in the antitumor effect of CPT-11. Cancer Res 1991; 51:4187-4191.

86. Kuchta RD, Willehlm L. Inhibition of DNA primase by 1-β-D-arabinofuranosyladenosine triphosphate. Biochem 1991; 30:797-803.

87. Perrino FW, Mekosh HL. Incorporation of cytosine arabinoside monophosphate into DNA at internucleotide linkages by human DNA polymerase α. J Biol Chem 1992; 267:23043-23051.

88. Bachur NR, Yu F, Johnson R et al. Helicase inhibition by anthracycline anticancer agents. Mol Pharmacol 1992; 41:993-998.

89. Bachur N, Johnson R, Yu F et al. Anti-helicase action of DNA binding anticancer agents: relationship to G/C intercalator binding. Mol Pharmacol 1993; 44:1064-1069.

90. Huang L, Turchi JJ, Wahl AF et al. Effects of the anticancer drug cis-diamminedichloroplatinum (II) on the activities of calf thymus DNA polymerase ε. Biochem 1993; 32:841-848.

91. Kufe DW, Major PP. Studies on the mechanism of action of cytosine arabinoside. Med Pediatr Oncol Suppl 1982; 1:49-67.

92. Glisson B, Gupta R, Smallwood-Kentro S et al. Characterization of acquired epipodophyllotoxin resistance in a chinese hamster ovary cell line: loss of drug-stimulated DNA cleavage activity. Cancer Res 1986; 46:1934-1938.

93. Yang L, Rowe TC, Liu LF. Identification of DNA topoisomerase II as an intracellular target of antitumor epipodophyllotoxins in simian virus 40-infected monkey cells. Cancer Res 1985; 45:5872-5876.

94. Ishimi Y, Ishida R, Andoh T. Effect of ICRF-193, a novel DNA topoisomerase II inhibitor, on simian virus 40 DNA and chromosome replication in vitro. Mol Cell Biol 1992; 12:4007-4014.

95. Tsao Y-P, Russo A, Nyamuswa G et al. Interaction between replication forks and topoisomerase I-DNA cleavable complexes: studies in a cell-free SV40 DNA replication system. Cancer Res 1993; 53:5908-5914.

96. Snapka RM, Permana PA. SV40 DNA replication intermediates: analysis of drugs which target mammalian DNA replication. BioEssays 1993; 15:121-127.

97. Pratt WB, Ruddon RW, eds. The anticancer drugs. New York: Oxford University Press 1979.

98. Chabner BA, Collins JM. Cancer chemotherapy: principle and practices. Philadelphia, PA: J.B. Lippincott Co. 1990.

99. Applegren N, Hickey RJ, Kleinschmidt AM et al. Further characterization of the human cell multiprotein DNA replication complex. J Cell Biochem 1995; 59:91-107.

CHAPTER 8

SV40 Circular Oligomer Series: Normal and Abnormal DNA Replication Intermediates

Robert M. Snapka and Paskasari A. Permana

The circular DNA genomes of bacteriophages and DNA viruses are usually thought of as having a unique size. However, cells infected or transformed by these viruses often contain small amounts of circular DNAs whose sizes are multiples of the unit (or monomer) genome (Fig. 8.1). The circular DNA oligomers consist of unit viral genomes joined covalently "head-to-tail." In contrast to the topologically linked catenated dimers ("chain-linked dimers," chapter 4), they are not intermediates in the replication of monomer genomes, but are separate pools of replicating circular DNAs. Multiple genome-length circular DNAs have been observed in cells infected with bacteriophages φX174,[1] P22,[2] and M13.[3] Cells transformed by a temperature-sensitive mutant of polyomavirus have been reported to produce circular dimers and trimers,[4] and circular oligomers of the SV40 genome have been found in lytically infected CV-1 (African green monkey kidney) cells.[5] Studies of circular oligomers have relied heavily on electron microscopy. Quantitation of circular oligomers by electron

The SV40 Replicon Model for Analysis of Anticancer Drugs,
edited by Robert M. Snapka. ©1996 R.G. Landes Company.

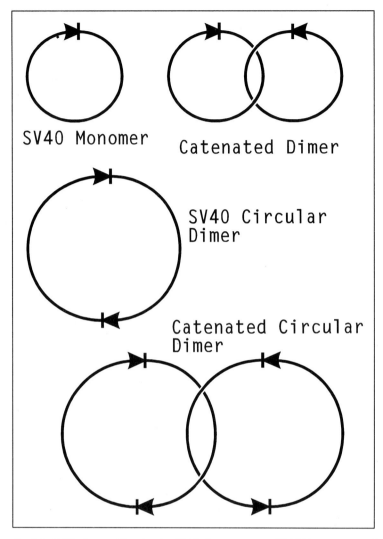

Fig. 8.1. SV40 dimers. The circular DNA chromosome of SV40 is represented by a circle. The vertical bar represents a randomly selected unique sequence such as the replication origin or a unique restriction endonuclease site. Catenated dimers are made up of two newly replicated SV40 daughter chromosomes which have not separated because they remain topologically linked. Although the two chromosomes making up a catenated dimer may be intertwined with one another over 25 times (catenation linking number > 25), catenation always involves dimers made up of two circular daughter chromosomes. A circular dimer is a single DNA circle composed of two SV40 chromosomes covalently joined "head-to-tail." Any unique SV40 DNA sequence, like the origin of DNA replication, occurs twice in a circular dimer. Since circular dimers can replicate, the daughter chromosomes may be topologically linked (catenated) after the completion of DNA replication. This would be a catenated circular dimer. In the same way, circular trimers and other circular oligomers can be catenated. A catenated trimer would be composed of two topologically linked DNA circles, each being made up of three SV40 sequences covalently joined head-to-tail.

microscopy is difficult, and identification is complicated by contaminating cellular DNA, overlap or contact of DNA ends from linear fragments and other potential artifacts. Unambiguous replication intermediates of the circular oligomers have not been demonstrated.

The order of circular oligomers in infected cells can be difficult to establish clearly. It is important because a monomer-dimer-trimer-tetramer (1-2-3-4...) series implies a different mechanism of origin than a monomer-dimer-tetramer-octamer (1-2-4-8...) series. A sister chromatid exchange during replication of a circular DNA gives rise to a double sized circle.[6] A sister chromatid exchange during replication of a monomeric genome would give a circular dimer. Another sister chromatid exchange during replication of the circular dimer would double the size again and produce a circular tetramer. A 1-2-4-8-series of circular oligomers would be expected from such a mechanism. There is some evidence that sister chromatid exchange may occur in SV40 DNA replication (chapter 3).

Several studies have suggested a 1-2-4-8 series or an origin by aberrant DNA replication for the SV40 circular oligomers. The observation that trimer-sized DNA circles were found in uninfected cells and mitochondria was interpreted to mean that the trimer-sized DNA circles in SV40-infected cells were, at least in part, mitochondrial DNA.[5] In another study, the SV40 circular trimer was reported to be significantly under-represented with respect to the other circular oligomers, and the trimer-sized circular DNA was estimated to be mostly mitochondrial DNA on the basis of infectivity data.[7] This was interpreted as favoring an origin of circular oligomers by rare events during DNA replication. Circular dimers and tetramers make up a significantly larger percentage of the SV40 DNA synthesized when protein synthesis was inhibited with cycloheximide.[8] This result favored an origin of circular oligomers by aberrant replication with monomers giving dimers and aberrant replication of dimers giving rise to tetramers.

A 1-2-3 series has also been reported for the SV40 circular oligomers.[9] This series might arise from excision of tandemly-arranged SV40 genomes integrated into cellular chromosomes,[4] rolling circle DNA replication,[10] or "onion-skin" DNA replication in which reinitiation occurs at the origin of replication before the first replication is completed.[11] An elegant experiment in which host cells were co-infected with two SV40 strains having different sized chromosomes ruled out the possibility that circular oligomers might arise by recombination between separate molecules, for instance a trimer produced by recombination between a monomer and a dimer.[12] Only homopolymers of the two different genomes were seen.

THE ORDER OF SV40 CIRCULAR OLIGOMERS

We have used high-resolution two-dimensional gel electrophoresis to study the SV40 circular oligomers with the idea that this new technology would be free of the artifacts and ambiguities which plague electron microscopy. The completely replicated forms of the circular dimer (forms I, II and III) are often evident as minor electrophoretic bands in experiments focused on replication of the monomeric genome. To visualize the higher circular oligomers (tetramers, pentamers, etc.) and their replication intermediates, it is necessary to carry out either longer electrophoretic separations or longer fluorographic exposures (or both). With the longer exposures, normal monomeric SV40 DNA replication intermediates tend to be overexposed. The circular oligomers are also easier to see in pulse-chase experiments in which radiolabel is chased into completely replicated forms by following tritiated thymidine pulse label with an excess of unlabeled thymidine (chapter 2). This greatly simplifies the pattern and prevents the weak circular oligomer bands from being obscured by replication intermediates of the lower members of the series.

Two different experiments were done to establish the order of the SV40 circular DNA oligomer series by gel electrophoresis. The first was based on the fact that the reciprocal of the electrophoretic mobility of double stranded linear DNA is a linear function of its size.[13] This relationship holds true over a wide range of agarose gel concentrations (0.4-2.8%) as long as the voltage is low (about 1.0 V/cm). The conditions of our standard first dimension agarose gel electrophoresis are well within these values (chapter 2). The completely replicated SV40 chromosomes were selectively labeled in a pulse-chase experiment in which the tritiated thymidine pulse label was chased with several changes of media containing an excess of unlabeled thymidine. The viral DNA was purified by Hirt extraction, proteinase K digestion, chloroform: isopropanol (24:1) extraction and ethanol precipitation. The vacuum-dried DNA pellet was taken up in loading buffer for the standard first dimension neutral agarose gel, mixed and added to a slot in the agarose submarine gel. Two-dimensional neutral-chloroquine agarose gel electrophoresis and fluorography (chapter 2) revealed the SV40 circular oligomer series (Fig. 8.2). In this long fluorographic exposure, a trace of intermediate Cairns structures (IC) can still be seen, and a dark smear connects the overexposed form I (superhelical) and form II (nicked circle) monomer bands. This vertical smear is a radiolytic DNA nicking artifact that is associated with heavily labeled form I bands. As the superhelical form I DNA moves through the first dimension gel, radiolytic decay causes DNA strand breaks which convert the superhelical DNA to nicked circular DNA. Loss of the compactness associated with superhelicity causes an immediate decrease in electrophoretic mobility. These newly created form II molecules migrate through the gel with the same electrophoretic mobility as those in the form II band, but remain ahead of that band due to their "head start" as form I molecules. Since the radiolytic nicking goes on throughout the time of the first dimension electrophoresis, these nicked molecules are distributed as an even smear between the form I and II bands. In the second dimension (chloroquine) electrophoresis, this smear of form II molecules migrates as form II. The result is an "L-shaped" figure in which the back of the form I band is connected to the form II band by a vertical stem.

The "L" pattern is repeated for each of the circular SV40 oligomers. Since each successive oligomer is a larger DNA, the electrophoretic mobility is reduced in both dimensions. The radiolytic nicking artifact can be used to identify the form II bands associated with each circular oligomer form I band. The circular dimer form III band has the same spatial relationship to the circular dimer form I and II bands that the monomer form III band has to the monomer form I and II bands. These form III bands are on a "smear" of label which extends from the origin of electrophoresis, through the mitochondrial DNA band, and on beyond the

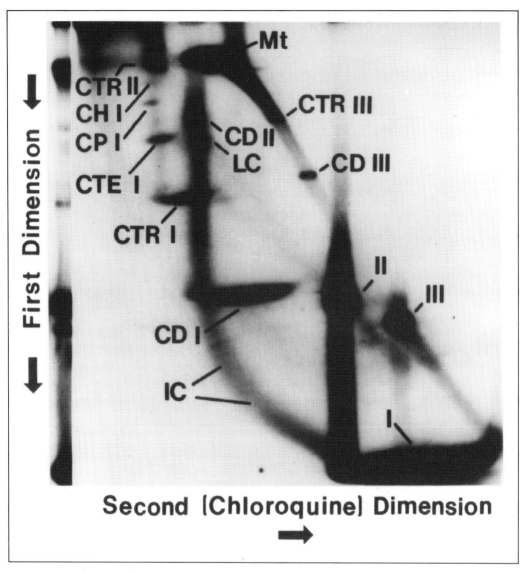

Fig. 8.2. Two-dimensional neutral-chloroquine gel electrophoresis of pulse-chased normal SV40 DNA replication intermediates. Abbreviations: Mt, mitochondrial DNA; I, form I (superhelical SV40 monomer); II, form II (nicked SV40 circle); III, form III (double strand linear SV40 DNA); IC, intermediate Cairns structures; CD I, form I circular (head-to-tail) dimer; CD II, form II circular dimer; CD III, form III circular dimer; CTR I, form I circular trimer; CTR II, form II circular trimer; CTR III, form III circular trimer; CTE I, form I circular tetramer, CP I, form I circular pentamer, CH I, form I circular hexamer. First dimension agarose gel electrophoresis was done from top to bottom as shown with a duplicated one dimensional gel, and second dimension gel electrophoresis in the presence of chloroquine was done from left to right as indicated. Details of the electrophoresis methods and structures of the major replication intermediates are discussed in chapter 2.

monomer form III band. This smear can be seen in Hirt extracted DNA from uninfected cells and consists of random length double stranded host cell DNA (mostly mitochondrial). All of the SV40 circular oligomer form III bands would be expected to appear on this smear. By varying the fluorographic exposure times, a series of form III bands for the SV40 circular oligomers can be seen, each corresponding to a form I and II band in the circular oligomer series.

The distance of each form III band from the first dimension origin of electrophoresis was plotted against the oligomer number for both a 1-2-3-4 series and a 1-2-4-8 series (Fig. 8.3). The relationship between the assumed oligomer number and the reciprocal of the electrophoretic mobility is only linear for the 1-2-3-4 series. On the basis of this result, the oligomers in Figure 8.2 were tentatively labeled as a 1-2-3-4 series. Assuming that these assignments are correct, the highest oligomer seen in Figure 8.2 is a circular hexamer.

The second experiment, done to confirm the assignments of the circular oligomer numbers, incorporated an artificial SV40 oligomer form III ladder. Completely replicated SV40 genomes were separated by neutral-chloroquine two-dimensional gel electrophoresis and compared on the same gel to a marker series of linear oligomers created by ligation of linearized form I molecules. Each replicating SV40 circular oligomer should have all three completely replicated forms (I, II and III). Comparison of the marker linear oligomers, a 1-2-3-series, with the corresponding SV40 circular oligomer form III bands gives the order of the circular oligomers. If there is a one-to-one correspondence, the order of the circular oligomers is 1-2-3. If only the even numbered marker form III bands have corresponding form III bands in the circular oligomers, the order of the circular oligomers is 1-2-4.

The markers were made by first labeling SV40 infected cells for 3 h (100 μCi/ml), purifying the DNA by Hirt extraction, proteinase K digestion, solvent extraction (chloroform: isopropanol, 24:1) and mini gel electrophoresis. The form I band was visualized by ethidium bromide fluorescence and was electrophoretically eluted. The eluted form I DNA was purified before digestion with EcoRI restriction endonuclease which makes a single double strand break (with overhanging ends) in the SV40 chromosome. After removal of the restriction endonuclease, the linearized DNA was ligated with T4 DNA ligase. Random ligation makes a 1-2-3-series of linear oligomers. While the linear marker DNA was being made, replicating SV40 genomes were labeled and prepared for electrophoresis. Replicating SV40 genomes were pulse-labeled with tritiated thymidine, and the label was then chased into completed

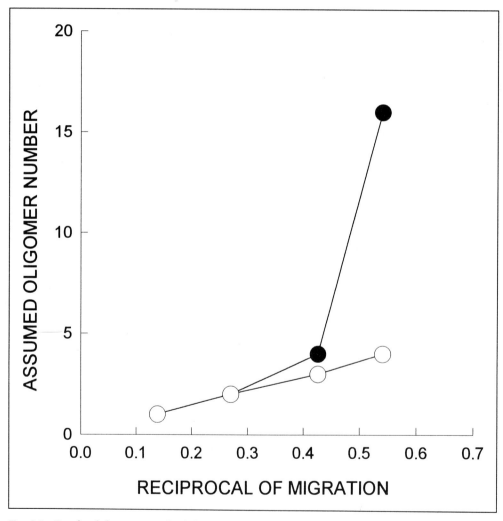

Fig. 8.3. Graph of the reciprocal of the first dimension electrophoretic migration versus assumed oligomer number for the form III bands of the circular oligomers. The data was obtained from an experiment similar to that shown in Figure 8.1. Assumed 1-2-4-8 series, ● ; assumed 1-2-3 series, ○.

forms by washing the cells several times in media with excess unlabeled thymidine. The viral DNA was prepared for electrophoresis and loaded into an agarose gel slot as described above for the
experiment shown in Figure 8.2. The linear marker DNA was
loaded several slots away on the same gel. In the first dimension
neutral agarose gel electrophoresis, the sample and the marker
DNAs ran parallel to one another but were separated by several
empty gel lanes. In the second dimension chloroquine gel electrophoresis, the markers migrated ahead of the replication
intermediates.

The resulting fluorograph (Fig. 8.4) shows the completed forms
(I, II and III) of the monomer, along with a trace of intermediate
Cairns structures. In this long fluorographic exposure, the vertical
smear discussed above can be seen connecting the form I and II
bands of each SV40 oligomer. Faint Keller bands can be seen to
extend from the right side of the form I monomer band. Only a
trace of the arc of monomer intermediate Cairns structure can be
seen.

The ligation of the linear marker DNA produced circular oligomers as well as linear oligomers. Thermal motion resulted in
low level superhelicity in the completely ligated circles. These are
resolved as Keller bands (K) in the first dimension electrophoresis.
The uppermost Keller band is covalently closed, but completely
relaxed form II DNA. Radiolytic nicking between the first and
second dimensions converted a small amount of each covalently
closed Keller band to a form II band. This is the origin of the
second set of bands below the partially ligated marker nicked circle
bands. In the presence of chloroquine, the covalently closed Keller
bands become positively supercoiled while the topology of their
nicked counterparts is unaffected. Keller bands can also be seen
for the marker DNA circular dimer, but Keller bands were not
resolved for higher circular oligomers of the marker DNA. Each
marker linear oligomer band is followed by a smear. Brief treatment with the single strand specific S1 nuclease before electrophoresis eliminates this smearing and causes the marker linear oligomers to migrate as sharp bands (P. Permana, unpublished data).
This suggests that the smearing of these bands is due to interactions

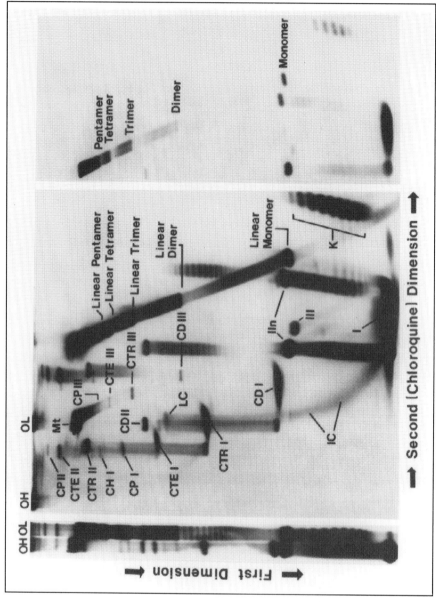

Fig. 8.4. Two-dimensional neutral-chloroquine gel electrophoresis of pulse-chased SV40 replication intermediates similar to that shown in Figure 8.1, but combined with a simultaneous separation of marker SV40 DNA made by ligating SV40 DNA that had been linearized by digestion with EcoRI. Abbreviations: K, Keller bands (covalently closed DNA circles with low level supercoiling); IIn, nicked circular DNA; LC, late Cairns structure; CP II, form II circular pentamer; OH, origin of electrophoresis for normal Hirt-extracted SV40 DNA replication intermediates (pulse-chased); OL, origin of electrophoresis for ligated SV40 DNA markers. Other abbreviations are the same as in Figure 8.1. The linear oligomers from the marker DNA are labeled linear monomer through linear pentamer. A shorter exposure of the right side of this gel is shown to the right to reveal the linear tetramer and pentamer more clearly.

between the single strand overhangs ("sticky ends") resulting from EcoRI digestion.

Comparison of the marker linear oligomers with the SV40 circular oligomer form III bands shows a one-to-one correspondence. This proves that the order of the SV40 circular oligomers is a 1-2-3 series and rules out an origin by sister chromatid exchange during normal viral DNA replication.

NORMAL AND ABERRANT REPLICATION INTERMEDIATES OF THE SV40 CIRCULAR OLIGOMERS

NORMAL REPLICATION INTERMEDIATES

Long fluorographic exposures of normal SV40 replication intermediates separated by two-dimensional gel electrophoresis reveal replication intermediates of the circular oligomers. In Figure 8.5, the arcs of the monomer, circular dimer and circular trimer intermediate Cairns structures can be seen on a two-dimensional neutral-chloroquine gel electrophoresis pattern. Since replication intermediates of the higher circular oligomers tend to be obscured by those of the lower circular oligomers, it is usually necessary to adjust fluorographic exposures carefully to see the replication intermediates of any particular circular oligomer. Although there is a possibility that a circular oligomer could have more than one replication bubble, it is likely to be an infrequent occurrence. The arcs of circular oligomer intermediate Cairns structures do not appear different in any way from those of the monomeric SV40 genomes.

CIRCULAR OLIGOMER CATENATED DIMERS

As discussed in chapters 2 and 4, inhibition of topoisomerase II causes accumulation of highly catenated SV40 chromosomes, each made up of two newly replicated daughter chromosomes which have not separated. The level of catenation can vary from one to more than 25. If each monomer making up a catenated dimer is superhelical, the dimer is a member of the C-family of catenated dimers. If both daughter chromosomes are nicked, the dimer is a member of the A-family. If one daughter chromosome is nicked and one is superhelical it is a B-family dimer. For the A- and

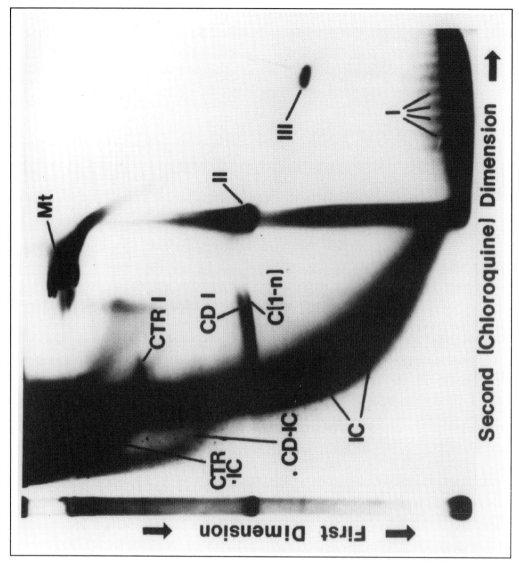

Fig. 8.5. Two-dimensional neutral-chloroquine gel electrophoresis of pulse-labeled SV40 DNA replication intermediates. A very long fluorographic exposure was used to demonstrate intermediate Cairns structure of the circular dimer and the circular trimer. Abbreviations: CD-IC, circular dimer intermediate Cairns structures; CTR-IC, circular trimer intermediate Cairns structures; C(1-n), C-family catenated dimers. Other abbreviations are the same as in Figure 8.1.

B-families of catenated dimers, each increase in catenation linking number causes a discrete increase in compactness and, thus, in electrophoretic mobility. One-dimensional agarose gel electrophoresis separates the A- and B-family catenated dimers into ladders of bands in which each band represents a specific level of catenation. The A- and B-dimer ladders overlap in the standard first dimension neutral agarose gel patterns (see chapter 2, Fig. 2.1).

Catenated dimers of the circular SV40 oligomers have never been evident in experiments involving inhibition of topoisomerase II. It is important to know if catenated circular dimers are present under these conditions. It has been suggested that the SV40 terminus region plays an important role in the formation of catenated dimers.[14,15] However, it has also been shown that termination of SV40 DNA replication occurs 180° from the origin of replication and does not require the normal terminal region DNA sequence.[16] In the circular SV40 dimer (and all even-numbered oligomers), another replication origin will be 180° from any other replication origin. If the terminus region is required for the formation of catenated dimers, topoisomerase II inhibition should not give rise to catenated circular dimers.

The absence of catenated circular dimers in experiments involving topoisomerase II inhibition may be more apparent than real. Even the completed forms of the circular dimers are normally very minor bands. As shown above, visualization of circular dimer replication intermediates requires long fluorographic exposures, and they tend to be obscured by replication intermediates of lower oligomers and monomers. Catenated circular dimers would also be expected to be distributed into three families of bands (A-, B- and C-families) like the catenated dimers of the monomeric viral chromosome. This distribution of the catenated dimers into three faint ladders of bands would make them even more difficult to detect.

Detection of catenated circular dimers requires simplification of the gel pattern. To eliminate the arcs of intermediate Cairns structures, infected cells were exposed to 40 μM proflavine for 30 min during labeling with tritiated thymidine. DNA intercalators like proflavine prevent the initiation of new rounds of SV40 DNA replication[17] and block the decatenation step of replication.[18] At the same time, proflavine does not greatly affect the flow of label out of early and intermediate Cairns structures. As with other topoisomerase II catalytic inhibitors, proflavine slows, but does not block the flow of label through the late Cairns structure.[18,19] A long exposure to proflavine during labeling causes most of the label to accumulate in catenated dimers. To further simplify the gel pattern, the purified SV40 DNA was kept at 4°C for 10 days so that extensive radiolytic nicking would convert the B- and C-family catenated dimers to A-family catenated dimers. Two-dimensional neutral-chloroquine agarose gel electrophoresis showed that the B- and C-families of catenated dimers had been almost completely converted to A-family catenated dimers by the radiolytic nicking (Fig. 8.6). A faint trace of highly catenated B-family dimers (MC) can be detected in this long fluorographic exposure. The intense A-family catenated dimer ladder makes a straight diagonal line of bands, as expected for a two-dimensional neutral-chloroquine gel pattern. A second line of finely spaced A-family catenated dimers extends upward from the ladder of monomer A-family dimer bands on the same diagonal. The monomer A-ladder extends well behind the position of the form II band to the position of the late Cairns structure and the form II circular dimer. The A1 catenated dimer, the late Cairns structure, and the form II circular dimer are all approximately double sized DNA circles. In the same way, this second ladder of bands extends well behind the form II circular dimer to the expected positions the form II circular tetramer and the circular dimer late Cairns structure. This evidence indicates that these bands represent A-family catenated circular dimers. This in turn shows that the terminus region is not necessary for the formation of catenated dimers when topoisomerase II is inhibited.

CIRCULAR OLIGOMER "40S" INTERMEDIATES

The DNA polymerase inhibitor aphidicolin causes replicating SV40 chromosomes to become torsionally stressed and very compact.[20,21] Recombinational events associated with the formation and breakdown of these 40S intermediates are discussed in chapter 3. We have asked if equivalent "40S-like" torsionally stressed replication intermediates occur in the SV40 circular oligomers when DNA

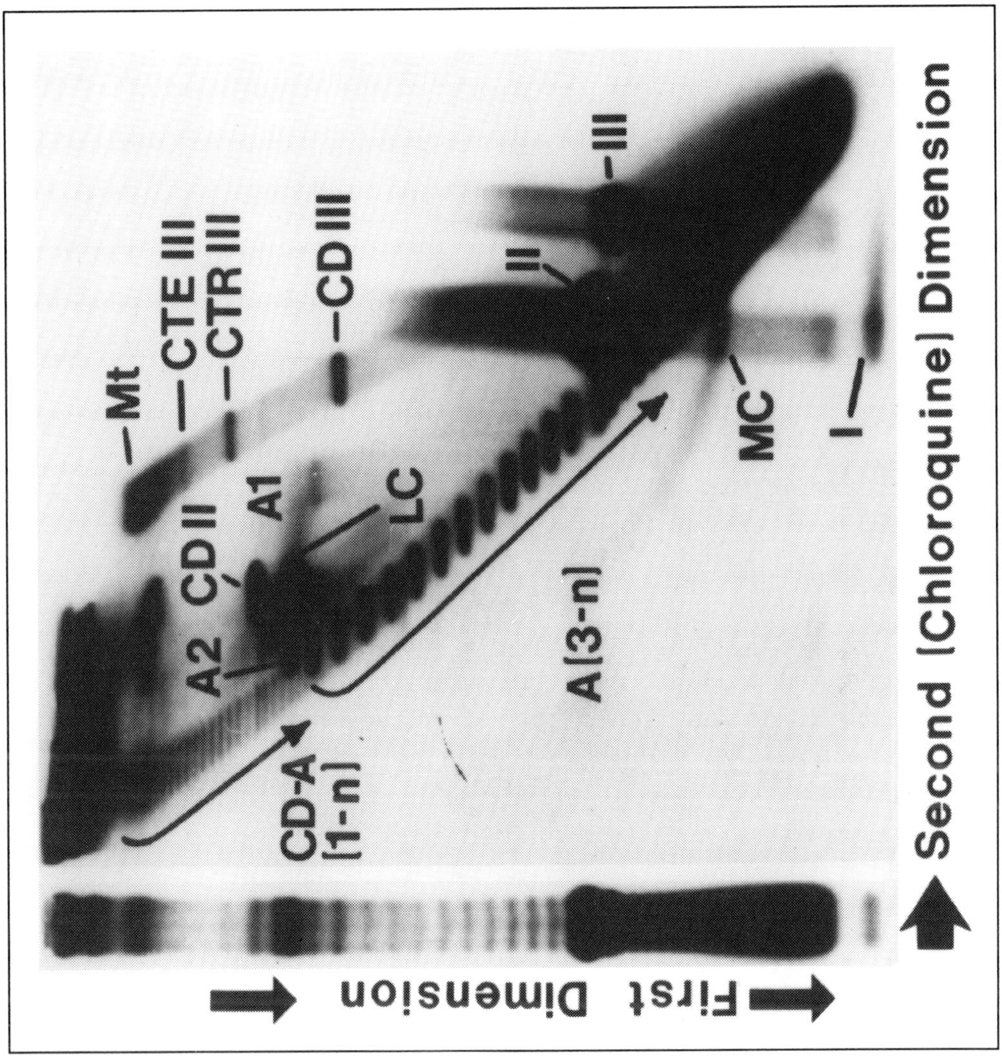

Fig. 8.6. Two-dimensional neutral-chloroquine gel electrophoresis of highly catenated A-family SV40 dimers resulting from exposure of infected cells to 40 μM proflavine. Extensive radiolytic DNA nicking was used to convert B- and C-family catenated dimers to A-family catenated dimers. Abbreviations: A1, singly catenated A-family dimer (composed of two monomeric SV40 DNA circles); A2, A-family catenated dimer with catenation linking number of 2; A(3-n), A-family catenated dimers with catenation linking numbers 3-n); CD-A(1-n), A-family catenated circular dimers with catenation linking numbers 1-n); MC, remnant of B-family dimers. MC is the point at which B-family dimers are no longer resolved. It appears as a pseudoband on one dimensional gel patterns. Other abbreviations are the same as in Figure 8.1.

replication is inhibited by aphidicolin. Of course, the equivalent torsionally stressed circular oligomer replication intermediates would not have a sedimentation coefficient of 40S. Since it is not possible to demonstrate circular oligomer replication intermediates by sucrose gradient ultracentrifugation, no sedimentation coefficient can be determined either for their normal intermediate Cairns structures or for torsionally stressed forms. For convenience, the torsionally stressed replication intermediates of circular oligomers will be called circular oligomer "40S" forms. Demonstration of similar circular oligomer "40S" intermediates was difficult because of the complexity of two-dimensional gel patterns in the higher molecular weight regions. Modifications of our standard two-dimensional gel systems gave indications of circular oligomer 40S intermediates, but they were not clear and unambiguous. An unusual approach was taken to simplify the gel pattern and demonstrated "40S" intermediates for the circular dimer and trimer.

In this experiment, normal SV40 DNA replication intermediates and aberrant intermediates resulting from exposure of the infected cells to aphidicolin were separated by two-dimensional neutral-chloroquine agarose gel electrophoresis. Between the first dimension electrophoresis and a second dimension chloroquine gel electrophoresis, the viral replication intermediates were denatured and then renatured by soaking the gel in alkaline then in neutral buffers. The results of this neutral-denaturation/renaturation-chloroquine two-dimensional gel electrophoresis are shown in Figure 8.7. The only pulse-labeled SV40 intermediates to renature were the form I superhelical chromosomes, including the monomer, the circular dimer, the circular trimer and the circular tetramer. Since the parental and daughter DNA strands in form I DNAs are both covalently closed and topologically intertwined, they cannot diffuse away from one another after denaturation. This topological linkage insures renaturation. The pulse-labeled nascent strands from other SV40 DNA replication intermediates were completely removed from the parental strands which are not labeled and do not contribute to the fluorographic image. The labeled full genome length nascent strands of the completely replicated forms II and III, not well resolved in the first dimension, migrated together as a single spot in the second dimension (labeled II).

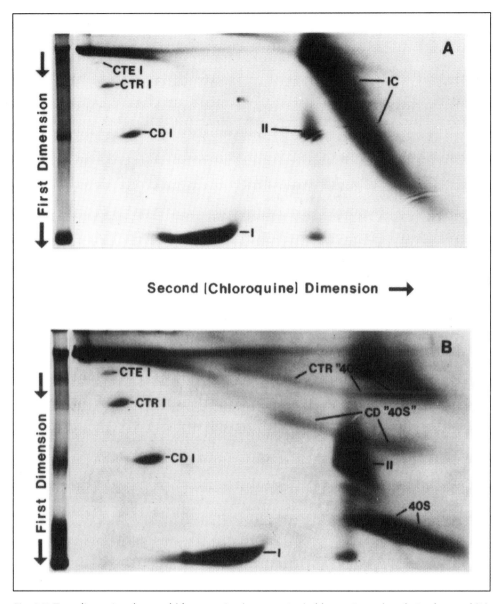

Fig. 8.7. Two-dimensional neutral-(denaturation/renaturation)-chloroquine gel analysis of normal (A) and "40S" intermediates (B) of the SV40 circular oligomers. Abbreviations: 40S, nascent strands from torsionally stressed 40S SV40 monomer replication intermediates; CD "40S"; torsionally stressed "40S-like" circular dimer DNA replication intermediates; CTR "40S", torsionally stressed "40S-like" circular trimer DNA replication intermediates. Other abbreviations are the same as in Figure 8.1.

The nascent strands from monomer SV40 intermediate Cairns structures (Fig. 8.7, A) range from very small to full genome length single strands and make an arc that stretches from the second dimension dye front to the position marked by the nascent strands from forms II and III. Most of the nascent strands from the circular dimer intermediate Cairns structures are included in this arc.

The electrophoretic pattern is very different for the SV40 DNA replication intermediates from cells treated with aphidicolin during DNA replication (Fig. 8.7, B). Exposure to aphidicolin causes the normal intermediate Cairns structures to become very compact and migrate as a thick band just behind the form I DNA band in the first dimension neutral gel electrophoresis (chapter 3). The nascent strands from these 40S intermediates form an arc that extends from the second dimension dye front to the position marked by the full length nascent strands from forms II and III. In contrast to the normal intermediates, this arc is greatly compressed in the first dimension. The same is true of the arcs of circular dimer and circular trimer "40S" intermediates which can be seen in the expected positions relative to their respective form I spots.

These experiments show that the SV40 circular oligomers are actively replicating and that their normal replication intermediates are indistinguishable from those of the monomeric SV40 chromosomes. Replication intermediates of circular oligomers up to the hexamer have been demonstrated by high-resolution two-dimensional gel electrophoresis of pulse-labeled viral DNA, and the sequence of circular oligomers has been proven to be a 1-2-3 series. This rules out an origin for the circular dimers by sister chromatid exchange during normal replication. An origin by excision of multimeric viral genomes integrated into cellular chromosomes is still a possibility. There is no evidence of rolling circle SV40 DNA replication intermediates in normal lytic infections, nor are there any unexplained forms which might be "onion skin" replication intermediates with multiple initiations at a single DNA replication origin. The absence of rolling circles or "onion skin" replication intermediates in the gel patterns does not rule them out as mechanisms for producing the circular oligomers. These replication forms could occur as rare events giving rise to a few circular oligomer molecules which would then have a replication advantage over monomeric viral chromosomes because of the increased number of replication origins.

These results are the first demonstration of intermediate Cairns structures of the circular oligomers and the first demonstration of aberrant SV40 circular oligomers resulting from exposure to drugs which inhibit enzymes of DNA replication. Inhibition of DNA polymerases and inhibition of topoisomerase II have the same effect on replicating SV40 circular oligomers that they have on the replicating monomer. These studies with the SV40 circular oligomers show the exceptional resolving power of two-dimensional gel electrophoresis and the many ways that it can be adapted to solve specific problems.

REFERENCES

1. Rush MG, Warner RC. Multiple-length rings of φX174 replicative form. II. Infectivity. Proc Natl Acad Sci USA 1967; 58:2372-2376.
2. Rhoades M, Thomas CA. The P22 bacteriophage DNA molecule. II. Circular intracellular forms. J Mol Biol 1968; 37:41-61.
3. Jaenisch R, Hofschneider PH, Preusa A. Isolation of circular DNA by zonal centrifugation. Separation of normal length, double length and catenated M13 replicative form DNA and of host specific episomal DNA. Biochim Biophys Acta 1969; 190:88-100.
4. Cuzin F, Vogt M, Dieckmann M et al. Induction of virus multiplication in 3T3 cells transformed by a thermosensitive mutant of polyoma virus. J Mol Biol 1970; 47:317-333.
5. Rush MG, Eason R, Vinograd J. Identification and properties of complex forms of SV40 DNA isolated from SV40-infected African green monkey (BSC-I) cells. Biochim Biophys Acta 1970; 228:585-594.
6. McClintock B. The production of homozygous deficient tissues with mutant characteristics by means of the aberrant behavior of ring shaped chromosomes. Genetics 1938; 23:315-376.
7. Jaenisch R, Levine A. DNA replication in SV40-infected cells. V. Circular and catenated oligomers of SV40 DNA. Virology 1971; 44:480-493.
8. Jaenisch R, Levine AJ. DNA replication in SV40-infected cells, VI. the effect of cycloheximide on the formation of SV40 oligomeric DNA. Virology 1972; 48:373-379.
9. Martin MA, Howley PM, Byrne JC et al. Characterization of supercoiled oligomeric SV40 DNA molecules in productively infected cells. Virology 1976; 71:28-40.

10. Goebel W, Helinski D. Generation of higher multiple circular DNA in bacteria. Proc Natl Acad Sci USA 1968; 61:1406-1413.

11. Botchan MW, Topp W, Stambrook J. Studies on SV40 excision from cellular chromosomes. Cold Spring Harbor Symp Quant Biol 1979; 43:709-719.

12. Rigby PWJ, Berg P. Does simian virus 40 DNA integrate into cellular DNA during productive infection? J Virol 1978; 28:475-489.

13. Southern EM. Preparative gel electrophoresis approaches for large scale separations. Anal Biochem 1979; 100:304-318.

14. Weaver DT, Fields-Berry SC, DePamphilis ML. The termination region for SV40 DNA replication directs the mode of separation for the two sibling molecules. Cell 1985; 41:565-575.

15. Fields-Berry SC, DePamphilis ML. Sequences that promote formation of catenated intertwines during termination of DNA replication. Nucleic Acids Res 1989; 17:3261-3274.

16. Lai C-J, Nathans D. Non-specific termination of simian virus 40 DNA replication. J Mol Biol 1975; 97:113-118.

17. Permana PA, Ferrer CA, Snapka RM. Inverse relationship between catenation and superhelicity in newly replicated simian virus 40 daughter chromosomes. Biochem Biophys Res Commun 1995; 201:1510-1517.

18. Snapka RM, Powelson MA, Strayer JM. Swiveling and decatenation of replicating simian virus 40 genomes in vivo. Mol Cell Biol 1988; 8:515-521.

19. Permana PA, Snapka RM, Shen LL et al. Quinobenoxazines: a class of novel antitumor quinolones and potent mammalian DNA topoisomerase II catalytic inhibitors. Biochemistry 1994; 33:11333-11339.

20. Dröge P, Sogo JM, Stahl H. Inhibition of DNA synthesis by aphidicolin induces supercoiling in simian virus 40 replicative intermediates. EMBO J 1985; 4:3241-3246.

21. Snapka RM, Shin C-G, Permana PA et al. Aphidicolin-induced topological and recombinational events in simian virus 40. Nucleic Acids Res 1991; 19:5065-5072.

INDEX

Items in italics denote figures (f) and tables (t).